VITALITY CHALLENGE

ART ULENE, MD

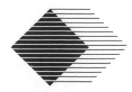

Published by: Black Diamond Associates
11340 West Olympic Boulevard, Suite 265
Los Angeles, CA 90064

Designed by: Media Content Marketing
405 Park Avenue, Suite 901
New York, NY 10022

ISBN: 0-9719025-0-x

Printed in the USA

TABLE OF CONTENTS

ACKNOWLEDGMENTS

The author gratefully acknowledges the contributions of:

- Walter Brackelmanns, MD, on whose ideas and clinical experience we have based the section on Relationships (Day 18).

- Bob Boone, MBA/MHA, CHE, President of the Medical Fitness Association, for his dedication to the betterment of public health and his strong support for The Vitality Challenge.

- Doug Clements, CSCS, NSCA-CPT, for his contributions to the section on Strength Training (Day 5).

- Joyce Deason, MS, CEP, for her contributions to the section on Aerobic Exercise (Day 4).

- Brian Lewis, PhD, for his contributions to the section on Flexibility (Day 2).

- Jamie McDowell, for her dedication, tireless efforts, and friendship.

- Joanne Pello, for her exceptional design skills and extraordinary patience.

- Neil Sol, PhD, for his thoughtful review and scientific contributions.

- Richard Trubo, for his skillful writing and tireless effort.

- Valerie Ulene, MD, for her professional contributions and comradeship.

- Kukla Vera, for the management skills and determination that put vitality into The Vitality Challenge.

- Hendrie Weisinger, PhD, on whose research and writing we have based the section on Managing Anger (Day 16).

- Cary Wing, EdD, Executive Director, MFA, for her support of The Vitality Challenge and her contributions to the section on Strength Training (Day 5).

INTRODUCTION

WHAT IS VITALITY?

Modern dictionaries contain several definitions for the word "vitality":..."*the capacity to live and develop*"..."*the power of enduring*"..."*the state of being alive.*" It doesn't take much—with those definitions—to qualify as a person with vitality.

I see vitality as a much grander state—the highest possible level of wellness. How can you tell if you have my kind of vitality? *Real* vitality? It's easy.

- If you wake up each morning feeling refreshed and looking forward to the day ahead—you have vitality.

- If you can briskly walk a mile or two, and still have energy for more—you have vitality.

- If you can meet the stress of daily life without *feeling* stressed— you have vitality.

- If you can eat all you want of foods you love and still not gain weight—you have vitality.

- If you can remain well while all around you are sneezing and sniffling—you have vitality.

- If you can argue without getting angry, and love without feeling fear—you have vitality.

What if you can do *all* of the things described above? Then you have *real* vitality, and you are *truly* alive. And you shouldn't settle for anything less. That's what the Vitality Challenge™ is all about.

THE VITALITY CHALLENGE

Many people assume that major sacrifices are necessary to attain such a high level of wellness. This attitude harks back to the now-discredited philosophy of "*no pain, no gain.*" But real vitality has nothing to do with pain or sacrifice; it comes from simple, easy lifestyle changes maintained consistently for long periods of time.

Real vitality involves a state of balance between all dimensions of wellness—not just the physical. You cannot overlook one aspect of your being without causing disharmony in others. All the strength in the world won't give you *real* vitality if you have ignored your nutritional, mental, emotional, spiritual, and medical needs. Losing twenty pounds won't make you feel good if you cough all the time from smoking. Walking two miles a day won't make you feel well if problems at work or home leave you feeling angry all the time. Meditating daily won't fill the gap if your diet is deficient in vitamins, minerals, proteins and fiber.

Life is different when you have developed *real* vitality. You feel balanced. You can live in a stressful world without feeling stressed. You actually get better as you grow older.

The program you are about to begin will guide you toward vitality in five critical areas: physical vitality, nutritional vitality, mental vitality, emotional and spiritual vitality, and medical vitality. Only by maintaining high levels of vitality in all of these areas can you achieve the *real* vitality described above. Now, let's define what we mean when we talk about "vitality" in each of these areas.

Physical Vitality

If you asked several people to define physical vitality, you would probably get several different answers, because each person looks at vitality or fitness in terms of his or her personal needs. A person who swims long distances wants stamina and endurance. Someone who does gymnastic routines requires flexibility. A middle-aged, sedentary person might be content with a slim waistline. The truth is, you can be extremely fit for one kind of task and completely out of shape for another.

Overall physical vitality is made up of three discrete components: aerobic fitness, muscle strength and joint flexibility. Each component of physical vitality provides a different benefit. Being aerobically fit will allow you to perform physically demanding work or engage in exercise for long periods of time without getting breathless, and it will decrease your risk of heart disease. Building muscle strength will enhance your balance and coordination, promote good posture and make your daily activities easier. Maintaining flexibility will protect your muscles and joints, relieve many aches and pains, and allow you to move about more comfortably.

To consider yourself physically fit, you must achieve a balance of fitness in each of these areas, and it takes different kinds of exercise to accomplish that. To develop aerobic fitness, you must exercise vigorously enough to raise your heart rate significantly. To build strength, you must make your muscles work against resistance. To promote flexibility, you need to stretch the connective tissues that bind your joints to their surrounding muscles. You will find more information about each of these areas later in the book, and the daily assignments will help you achieve a balance in all three areas.

Nutritional Vitality

There are many different ways to look at nutritional vitality. Some people assume they are nutritionally fit if their weight is in the desired range. (Ironically, many of these same people have severe nutritional deficiencies because of the fad diets they use to keep their weight in that range.) Others think they are nutritionally fit because they use vitamin and mineral supplements (at the same time their diets are filled with fatty foods that are low in fiber). Some individuals seek nutritional vitality by avoiding certain food categories, like meat or dairy products (and fail to make up for the iron or calcium that these categories provide so well).

The truth is, there is no single diet that will meet everyone's nutritional needs. While some people need to severely restrict the amount of fat and cholesterol in their diet, others may safely tolerate larger amounts. And while some people must restrict the amount of salt in their diet because it raises their blood pressure, others do not respond this way and can tolerate larger amounts without jeopardizing their health. And a young, thin athlete who exercises intensely for hours every day requires far more calories than a sedentary person who is overweight.

But there are some general nutritional principles that apply to everyone:

Real foods are your best source of vitamins and minerals. A varied and balanced diet is the best way to ensure that your body is provided with the essential nutrients you need for good health. Foods provide you with other important substances that you can't get from pills, including flavonoids and other so-called phytochemicals that appear to play an important role in the prevention of cancer and other diseases. Foods also provide proteins, carbohydrates and essential fatty acids, without which your body cannot function normally. And foods provide fiber, which promotes healthy intestinal function and can reduce your risk of high blood cholesterol, heart disease and colon cancer.

That doesn't mean that vitamin and mineral supplements should not be used to reach optimal levels of intake for certain nutrients. Just keep in mind this fact: A poor diet plus supplements is still a poor diet.

Drastic dietary changes produce dangerous nutritional deficiencies. It is not possible to cut back drastically on your caloric intake or your intake of any major food category without jeopardizing your intake of certain nutrients. That's because nature did not distribute all nutrients equally in all foods. Dairy products are exceptionally rich in calcium; meats are exceptionally rich in iron; and dietary fiber is found exclusively in plant foods. That's why it's so important to avoid severely restrictive diets that promise radical benefits, such as rapid weight loss. These diets also deliver radical risks. The program you are about to begin does not require any drastic reductions of energy intake or of any particular food category that could result in a deficiency of important nutrients.

The goal of nutrition is not just to keep you alive and prevent deficiency diseases, but to help you achieve optimal health and *real* vitality. For decades—and even today— most nutritional recommendations have been based on the lowest level necessary to prevent deficiency symptoms, with a modest margin of safety added. The scientific panel that sets the RDAs for vitamins and minerals states that its recommendations are based on the amount that should "be adequate to meet the known nutrient needs of practically all healthy persons." But what if you're not healthy? And what do they mean by "practically all"? Who is left out by their definition?

Those RDAs may be much too low for people who have medical disorders such as diabetes or kidney disease, people who use alcohol or certain medications, and those who have unusual dietary patterns. Also, there is evidence now that larger doses of at least some nutrients can do far more than simply prevent deficiency diseases. To the extent that you can potentially benefit from larger doses, it makes sense to increase your consumption—provided the monetary cost is reasonable and the potential risk of adverse reactions is low. For this reason, you will find some recommendations in this book that exceed the current RDAs.

Mental Vitality

It is not possible to live in today's hectic world without encountering stressful situations. But that doesn't mean you have to let the stress make you sick. When you are mentally fit, you can recognize your sources of stress, and develop procedures to reduce their frequency and intensity. When stress can't be avoided, if you are mentally fit you can use techniques that cancel its ill effects.

What happens when you are not mentally fit? You ignore the stress. Before long, your heart pounds, your blood pressure rises, your hormones surge, you can't sleep. These are natural responses to stress, and they won't hurt you unless they happen all the time. Then the pounding becomes palpitations, the rapid pulse becomes a tachycardia, the rise in blood pressure becomes hypertension, sleeping difficulties become insomnia. The natural response to stress becomes disease.

In our program, you will learn how to identify your sources of stress and what you can do to eliminate some of them. You will never be able to get rid of all outside stress, but we'll show you how to manage the remaining stress more comfortably. With practice, you'll learn how to turn external stress into a positive force for change.

Emotional and Spiritual Vitality

Have you ever noticed that some of the most "fit" people you meet are also some of the unhappiest? These are people who have achieved high levels of fitness in one of the categories we've described, but who have neglected their emotional and spiritual needs. In spite of their accomplishments in one dimension of fitness, life holds no joy for them, and they look forward with despair to growing older.

Contrast these people with the ones you know who can't wait to see what the future holds for them—people who truly believe that life gets better every year.

Why does life get better for them? Because they get better at living life. They have personally meaningful goals and they know how to achieve them. They learn to change loneliness into serenity and feelings into action. They learn to express anger as well as affection, to live with a plan as well as to be spontaneous. They know how to satisfy the many different and conflicting needs of their own personality.

These people prove that learning doesn't stop when you leave school, growing doesn't stop when you finish puberty, and life doesn't end when you leave your youth. They teach us that the best part of life lies ahead—if we are willing to change as life changes. They show us that *real* vitality cannot be achieved without emotional and spiritual fitness.

The program you are about to begin will show you how to enhance your emotional and spiritual fitness level. You'll find information on how to improve your relationships with others, and assignments that get you started on the process. We'll show you new ways for managing anger without hurting yourself or the people around you, and we'll give you assignments that let you practice these techniques. You'll learn about the effect that altruism and social connections can have on health, and you'll do assignments that demonstrate the effect of these elements on your health. And you'll examine—and reexamine—the priorities that influence not just your behavior, but who you really are.

Medical Vitality

We have invented this unique fitness category to cover the preventive medical activities you can do to minimize your risk of illness and accidents. This category includes some obvious medical procedures, like immunizations and screening tests, and some less apparent (and less medical) activities like using seat belts and wearing bicycle helmets. A person who is "medically fit" (using our definition) has taken advantage of every preventive measure that is appropriate in his or her particular case.

We think it's important to include this category in any definition of *real* vitality, because people who are medically fit have a much lower risk of illness, disability and death than those who ignore these opportunities for protection. There's a dramatic difference in the injury and death rates of auto accident victims who use seat belts all the time and those who don't; and between cyclists who wear helmets every time they ride and those who don't. And there's a great difference in the hospitalization and mortality rates of older people who are immunized against influenza and pneumonia and those who are not.

The same substantial differences can be demonstrated for people who are medically screened at appropriate intervals and those who are not. Women who are screened for breast cancer at appropriate intervals have a significantly better survival rate than women who ignore mammography. (Women who are screened are also more likely to be eligible for breast-conserving surgery.) Women who are screened at appropriate intervals with Pap smears have almost no chance of dying of cervical cancer, yet nearly 5,000 women die of this disease every year in the United States—almost all of them because they failed to get Pap smears. Even "simple" screening tests, like blood pressure measurements and blood cholesterol determinations, can make a huge difference, because they permit the detection of potential problems many years before any serious damage is done.

During the next four weeks, you'll learn what you can—and should—do to make yourself medically fit. Several days in the program are actually dedicated to this aspect of fitness, and on those days you will find information about a wide range of preventive activities. After reviewing this information, especially the sections on immunizations and screening, talk to your own physician to determine which of the guidelines are appropriate in your particular case. Then work with your physician and do whatever else is necessary to complete those assignments appropriately.

HOW DO YOU ACHIEVE *REAL* VITALITY?

The process of achieving *real* vitality begins with recognizing the opportunity for improvement and making a commitment to change. If you do not believe that the quality of your life could be improved, and if you are not committed to at least attempting some change, there is no point in reading further, because simply reading—this book or any other—can't make you fit. If all it took to make people healthier was reading a book, we'd be the healthiest people in the world (and the thinnest, considering the number of diet books that have been sold).

If you want to achieve *real* vitality, you have to do it for yourself. You have to start caring *about* yourself and caring *for* yourself. That doesn't mean you have to exercise to the point of pain, or give up all the food you love to eat, or maintain the lifestyle of a saint. *Real* vitality doesn't require that you shut yourself away from all stressful situations or master the art of meditation. On the contrary, you can eat delicious foods without guilt; enjoy physical activities without discomfort; and confront stressful situations without getting sick. Your entire life actually gets better, because *you* are getting better in all dimensions of your being.

This book will provide the information and structure you need to reach the goal of *real* vitality. The book contains scientific information that will help you understand what is needed to achieve your goal. It also includes a highly structured 28-day program of assignments to get you on the right path.

Will you be *really* fit—totally fit—if you follow the program for 28 days? Probably not, unless you are very close to that point now. But I can promise you this: If you do every assignment for the next 28 days, you will learn the process of building vitality, and that is far more important than reaching your goal in four weeks. *Real* vitality is a lifetime process of continuing self-evaluation and constant self-improvement. It's a pleasurable process that leads to a lifetime of pleasure.

What about the other promises this book makes: an inch off your waist, a minute off your mile, 10 points off your blood pressure, 10 percent off your cholesterol level and fewer aches and pains. If you really do have room to improve in each of those areas, and you do all the assignments, those promises can be fulfilled in 28 days. But you shouldn't limit your vision of this program to the achievement of those finite goals. Our ultimate goal—and our ultimate promise—is to give you a sense of control over your life and confidence in your ability to achieve and maintain *real* vitality for the rest of your life.

Now it's time for you to make a promise: That you will follow this program as closely as you can for the next 28 days. The program in this book is only as good as your promise to follow it. If you are ready to make that promise, it's time to get started.

SELF-ASSESSMENT QUESTIONNAIRE

As you get started on the Vitality Challenge program, it is important to assess where you now stand. So spend a few minutes filling out the following *Self-Assessment Questionnaire.* The answers to these questions will give you a clear picture of your overall fitness level today, and will help you identify those areas in which you most need to improve. Write your answers directly on the questionnaire itself.

NAME: _____ TODAY'S DATE: _____

HEIGHT: _____ WEIGHT: _____ WAIST: _____

TOTAL CHOLESTEROL: _____ HDL: _____

LDL: _____ (*if total cholesterol is elevated*)

BLOOD PRESSURE: _____

TIME ELAPSED WALKING OR RUNNING A MEASURED MILE (*see page 57 for instructions on how to properly determine this time*): _____

1. Do you currently engage in aerobic exercise (any physical activity that is sufficiently intense to raise your heart rate during the period of exercise without making you feel "breathless") on a regular basis?   yes   no

    What activity or activities do you usually do? _____

    _____

    _____

    How many times per week do you typically engage in aerobic exercise?
            0   1 or 2   3 or 4   5 or 6   every day

2. Do you regularly do stretching exercises?   yes   no
    If so, how many times per week?
            0   1 or 2   3 or 4   5 or 6   every day

3. Do you do any strength training?   yes   no
    If so, how many times per week?
            0   1 or 2   3 or 4   5 or 6   every day

4. Rate the amount of fat in your diet:

     very low in fat   somewhat low-fat   lightly reduced in fat
     (approx. 10%)   (approx. 20%)   (approx. 30%)

        typical American diet   very high-fat
        (approx. 34% fat)   (over 35% fat)

5. Rate the amount of salt (sodium) in your diet:

_____ Very low (*I am careful about the packaged foods I eat and never add salt at the table or during cooking.*)

_____ Moderate (*I do not add salt at the table, but I am not particularly careful about packaged foods.*)

_____ Heavy (*I add salt at the table and do not monitor my salt intake in any way.*)

6. How many half-cup portions of fruits and vegetables do you usually eat in a day?

     0   1-2   3-4   5-6   7 or more

7. Do you have a clear list of priorities and a conscious plan of action that is designed to help you get what you want out of life—including your work life, your family life, and your friendships?

_____ No, I've really never thought of this in a concrete way.

_____ Sort of. While I have thought of it, I have never structured a specific plan with real goals and dates attached to it.

_____ Yes, I have a real plan and I actively put it to use. (*If you checked this response, briefly describe the top three priorities in your life.*)

1. _____

2. _____

3. _____

8. How often do aches and pains disrupt your life?

never   once a week   a few times a week   many times a week   every day

9. How actively do you try to meet the Recommended Daily Allowances (USRDAs) for vitamins and minerals?

    _____ I do not know the USRDAs, and I make no active attempt to monitor or meet any particular nutrient needs.

    _____ I am aware of the USRDAs, but I make no active attempt to monitor or meet any particular nutrient needs.

    _____ I am aware of the USRDAs, and I attempt to meet my nutrient needs through my diet.

    _____ I am aware of the USRDAs, and I attempt to meet my nutrient needs through the use of vitamin and mineral supplements.

    _____ I am aware of the USRDAs, and I attempt to meet my nutrient needs through my diet and the use of supplements.

10. How often do you have trouble sleeping?

never	almost never	once a week	a few times a week	almost always	always

11. How often do you awaken feeling refreshed and rested?

never	almost never	once a week	a few times a week	almost always	always

12. How stressed do you feel in general?

    _____ I often have more stress than I can bear.

    _____ My stress is bearable, but still taxing on me physically and mentally.

    _____ There is considerable stress in my life, but it is not taxing me physically or mentally.

    _____ There is little stress in my life, and I am able to handle it well.

    _____ I have no stress in my life.

13. How often do you use stress management techniques or relaxation techniques (such as meditation, self-hypnosis or imagery) to counter the effects of the stress in your life?

    never   almost   once   a few times   almost   always

                never   a week   a week   always

14. If there is a "significant other" in your life, how happy are you with that relationship?

    extremely   happy   satisfied   somewhat   unhappy

      happy   dissatisfied

15. Have you volunteered your time or money to a good cause in the last year?

                                       yes   no

16. Do you drink alcoholic beverages?   yes   no

If yes, how often do you drink:

    every day   a few times a week   once a week   less frequently

When you drink, how much do you drink?

    1 drink   2 drinks   3 drinks   more than 3 drinks

17. Why do you drink? (*Check all appropriate answers*)

_____ I like the flavor and/or thirst-quenching properties of the beverage.

_____ Drinking relaxes me.

_____ Drinking makes it easier for me to socialize.

_____ Drinking brings out my personality.

_____ Drinking helps me tolerate my life.

18. Overall, how do you feel about your life?

    extremely   happy   satisfied   somewhat   unhappy

      happy   dissatisfied

EVALUATING YOUR RESPONSES

Now, take a moment to review your responses on this questionnaire. What do they tell you about your *real* vitality level? Is there a balance among all of the different categories, or have you neglected some important areas? Remember: You cannot mistreat one aspect of your being without causing disharmony in others. Ignore one of your parts and something goes wrong with another.

- If everyone at home makes you tense and angry, running three miles a day won't produce a state of vitality. Running may help you release some of the tension and anger, but these feelings will keep returning unless you work on improving your relationships. You'll find some techniques in our program that can help you improve them.

- If you cough all the time from smoking, losing twenty pounds won't result in *real* vitality. Taking off the excess weight may help you look better, and it will improve some aspects of your health, but you'll never feel *really* fit as long as nicotine is constricting your coronary arteries and cancer-causing chemicals and tars are irritating the lining of your breathing passages.

- If unresolved conflicts from your past are constantly stirring up your emotions, meditating regularly won't create a sense of vitality. Enjoying meditation in a tension-provoking world is a great idea, but learning to recognize and deal successfully with the root causes of your unhappiness is the only way to keep those distressing feelings from interfering with your life.

What did you learn about yourself from the questionnaire? Take a moment to reflect upon what your answers mean. Perhaps you've singled out one or two specific areas that need your attention most. However, as the program gets underway, and you learn about all the factors that contribute to your vitality, you may find that you have more work to do than you initially thought.

No matter what your answers show, however, remember that this is an *overall* vitality program, not one that focuses on just a single category of wellness. You'll find a holistic approach in this book, which means that *every* component of the plan is important, and capable of contributing to your enhanced well-being. I hope you will take advantage of all of it .

HOW TO USE THIS BOOK

The remainder of this book contains a 28-day program designed to produce the comprehensive kind of *real* vitality that was described in the *Introduction*. Each day covers a specific subject or issue that is important to the process of developing overall vitality. On Day 1, for example, you'll read about dietary fat. On Day 2, about flexibility…and so on. Each day you will be provided with scientific information about the specific subject and with detailed assignments that relate to the topic.

Occasionally, the specific topic for the day may not be relevant to your particular fitness or medical needs. For example, Day 16 deals with anger, and angry outbursts may not be a problem in your life. Read the section anyway, even if the issue does not seem to apply directly to you. Covering the material may help you better understand why some around you behave the way they do. You may also be surprised that you can learn something about yourself, too, in the process.

Each of the 28 days also contains a series of specific assignments to do that day. Some of the assignments are keyed to the featured topic of the day; others relate to subjects previously discussed. To get the full fitness benefits from this carefully structured plan, you must do all of these assignments as diligently as possible, unless your physician has advised you against these activities because of your particular medical circumstances.

PACING YOURSELF

As you will soon see, some of the assignments appear very modest. For example, on Day 1 you will be asked to walk one mile. Each day thereafter, you'll be asked to speed up your walking time by just two to three seconds. That may not sound like very much, but cutting your time by two more seconds every day—day after day—soon adds up. By the end of 28 days, you'll be walking the same mile one minute faster, and you'll be able to do it without getting winded.

You may be tempted to increase our assignments so you can progress more rapidly toward your goal. In general, we'd like to discourage you from doing this, in part to ensure your safety, and partly because we want to make the process of change as easy and comfortable as we can for you. This approach works best over the long term, because it allows you to change without pain or discomfort, and without feeling like you are being deprived of something important to you.

The assignments also build upon one another—that is, there is a synergistic effect among them. Each one gains strength from the others, and by the time this multifaceted program becomes fully integrated into your life, their impact begins to multiply. As you add each new activity to those you've already made part of your life, the overall effect is quite impressive.

You can start the program on any day of the week, although you may find it a little easier to start on a Monday, since two days of each seven-day sequence in the book are laid out as "weekend days." On these days, you will find the same kind of assignments as on other days, but there will be no new featured topics to read. Use this time to play "catch-up," reviewing any sections you may not have had enough time to read carefully the first time around.

MONITORING YOUR PROGRESS

Research shows that a technique called "self-monitoring" can significantly increase the likelihood that you will reach your goal. This process simply involves a daily review of your goals and activities, followed by some form of written entry into an ongoing record. Careful monitoring and recording of your activities will reveal what you are doing right and in which areas you need to improve.

There are many different systems for monitoring and recording your progress, ranging all the way from detailed diaries to complex wall posters. Some people in fitness programs find these systems to be extremely helpful; others find them too burdensome to fit into their already busy schedules.

The system you will use to monitor and record your progress for the next 28 days is a simple and uncomplicated approach that forces you to think about what you are doing each day in the five key fitness areas of our program: Physical Vitality, Nutritional Vitality, Mental Vitality, Emotional and Spiritual Vitality, and Medical Vitality.

At the end of each day, take a few moments to evaluate and record how you performed on your specific assignments for the day. As shown in the key, use a pencil or pen to fill in the entire circle if you fully accomplished a particular assignment. Fill in just half the circle if you completed only part of the goal. And if you had a bad day with respect to that component of the program, leave the circle completely empty.

Keep in mind that you will be making general, qualitative evaluations of how you're doing. Try to reach fair and realistic judgments of how well you're doing, and then record those evaluations on the chart. Each day, as you are filling in the circles that chart your progress, ask yourself not just "What did I do today?" but also "Why?" As you answer the question "why," you will begin to recognize the specific problems that undermine your *real* fitness efforts. Then you can make adjustments in your daily routine that will help you deal effectively with those issues.

Filling in your assignment chart—and, more specifically, analyzing it—will enable you to learn what helps and hinders you and to put that knowledge into future plans and action. Think of your daily assignment charts as visual portraits of your fitness activities in the different categories. At a glance, these charts can reveal how you are doing generally, and identify specific areas where you need to begin concentrating more attention.

Each time you review your assignment charts during the next 28 days, see whether you can detect patterns that are creating problems for you. If many empty or half-empty circles appear on the assignment pages during a particular week, if they appear repeatedly on a particular day of the week, or if they appear repeatedly in the same assignment category, ask yourself why this is happening. The answer to that simple question may help you pinpoint particular situations or emotions that are triggering problems.

Self-monitoring is not just about finding your weaknesses and problem areas. It is just as useful for highlighting your strengths in this program. As you look closely at days when you've done very well, ask yourself what you can learn from those experiences. How can you apply the strategies that brought you success in those situations to other areas in which you still might be having problems?

Remember, self-monitoring is a dynamic process. Filling in the circles on the assignment pages is just the first step. You need to feed the information you gain from monitoring and charting back into your program, using it as a springboard for the next day's efforts. Your efforts will be repaid with even greater progress in the future.

THE USE OF TOBACCO PRODUCTS, IN ANY FORM, IS INCOMPATIBLE WITH *REAL* VITALITY. IF YOU SMOKE OR YOU ARE USING OTHER TOBACCO PRODUCTS, IT IS ESSENTIAL THAT YOU DISCONTINUE THIS PRACTICE BEFORE STARTING THE VITALITY CHALLENGE. DO NOT PROCEED WITH THE PROGRAM UNTIL YOU HAVE DONE THAT.

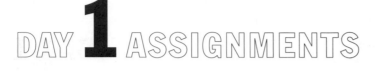

DAY **1** ASSIGNMENTS

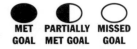

MET GOAL   **PARTIALLY MET GOAL**   **MISSED GOAL**

PHYSICAL VITALITY

1. Time your speed over a measured mile.   **Time:**_____
   (For instructions on measuring your mile, see box on page 57.)

NUTRITIONAL VITALITY

2. Count the total number of fat grams you consumed today.

3. Eat at least 7 half-cup portions of fruits and vegetables.

MENTAL VITALITY

EMOTIONAL & SPIRITUAL VITALITY

MEDICAL VITALITY

FAT   DAY 1

Fat is an essential nutrient in the diet. It provides part of the energy your body needs to keep running, and it is necessary for the absorption of certain vitamins (A, D, E and K). Fat plays a critical role in normal brain development in babies, and certain kinds of fat may actually protect you against disease. However, eating too much fat can be bad for your health. Excessive fat consumption can:

- **Increase your risk of cardiovascular disease.** Fats (particularly saturated fats) are converted into cholesterol by your body and can cause your blood cholesterol level to rise, which increases your risk of developing coronary heart disease and suffering a heart attack. High-fat diets also contribute to the development of obesity, which in turn increases your risk of diabetes and high blood pressure—both of which are risk factors for heart disease and stroke.

- **Increase your risk of cancer.** High-fat diets can increase the risk of certain cancers, particularly cancer of the colon, breast and prostate. High-fat diets also contribute to obesity, which increases the risk of cancer of the uterus. Animal fat, in particular, is a problem. Harvard researchers who studied 122,000 nurses for several years found that those who ate beef, lamb or pork each day had more than twice the risk of developing colorectal cancer as those who didn't eat red meat. High-fat, low-fiber diets slow the movement of waste material through the colon, which increases the exposure of the bowel to potentially cancer-causing substances.

HOW LOW SHOULD YOU GO?

The average American consumes about 34 percent of his or her daily calories as fat. That's an improvement from the 37 percent level of the mid-1980s and the 45 percent level of the mid-60s—but still far above the levels consumed in some undeveloped societies, where the rates of obesity, heart disease and stroke are so much lower than in the U.S.

The American Heart Association, the American Cancer Society, and the National Cholesterol Education Program recommend that you limit your fat intake so it accounts for no more than 30 percent of your total calories each day. But many experts challenge this recommendation because they feel it doesn't go far enough—especially for people who have a problem with high blood cholesterol or an elevated risk of coronary heart disease.

The Pritikin program, which received worldwide attention in the 1970s and 1980s, actually got fat intake down near five percent. And the heart diet leader of the 1990s, Dr. Dean Ornish of the University of California at San Francisco, has reduced his patients' fat consumption to 10 percent—with remarkable results. In people who follow the Ornish program—10 percent fat and very little dietary cholesterol (about 5 milligrams a day)—total cholesterol levels plummet a startling 24 percent.

Perhaps even more significantly, Ornish's program produced another impressive achievement: reversing blockage in the coronary arteries (the vessels that supply blood to the heart muscle). After one year on his program (which consisted of a low-fat diet, moderate exercise, smoking cessation and stress management), 82 percent of the patients in his study had reversed—at least in part—the process of atherosclerosis that was clogging their arteries. And they accomplished this reversal of the disease without the use of prescription medications. (For more about Ornish's research, see Day 10.)

FAT RESTRICTION IN CHILDREN

Children under the age of two should not be placed on a fat-restricted diet. At this age, abundant amounts of dietary fat are needed for normal development of the brain and nervous system and to meet the high energy needs of growing children. After the age of two, a reduced-fat diet may be appropriate for some children, but such a diet should be instituted only in consultation with the child's pediatrician.

In 2001, the National Heart, Lung, and Blood Institute reported on its long-term study showing that children with high blood cholesterol levels can benefit from a reduced-fat diet without interfering with their normal growth or sexual maturation during puberty.

In the past, I have generally recommended a diet that gets 20 percent of its calories from fat—halfway between the generous guidelines of the Heart Association and Cancer Society and the fairly rigid plans developed by Mr. Pritikin and Dr. Ornish. This diet is easy to follow, and it usually produces excellent results for most people who want to lose weight or need to reduce their blood cholesterol levels.

However, for people who want to achieve real vitality, I've got to agree with Pritikin and Ornish: 10 percent is better. So a reduction of your fat consumption to 10 percent is the goal I'll ask you to achieve during the next four weeks. If you are used to consuming large amounts of fat, this goal may not be easy. Fat tastes good, it makes food feel good in your mouth, and it's difficult to give up—at first. I know that from first-hand experience. But I also know that once you get your fat level down to 10 percent, you won't want to go back up. And once you learn how to substitute other sources of moisture and flavor for the fat you've been eating, you'll feel like you're eating better than ever.

HOW TO KEEP TRACK

There are two ways to stay focused on the fat target:

The law of averages: One approach is to let the "law of averages" get you to your goal of 10 percent fat calories. It's the same law you use when driving your car. (If half your drive is spent at 35 miles per hour and the other half is spent at 55 miles per hour, you don't need fancy calculations to know that your average speed for the trip will be 45.)

The same thing is true when you're dealing with the fat content of your diet. If you eat as much as you can of foods that are nonfat or very close to it, and you eat little or no food that is higher than 20 percent fat, the law of averages will keep your total fat intake somewhere around the 10 percent level. Even if you eat a couple of slices of bacon (about 80 percent fat calories) or a scoop of ice cream (about 50 percent fat calories) or a small pat of butter (100 percent fat calories), the law of averages will be on your side if you eat mostly nonfat and very low-fat foods the rest of that day. Reducing your fat is that simple.

Using this approach means you don't need a rigid menu plan, and there won't be any foods that are absolutely forbidden. You just have to balance out your high-fat choices with some good, very low-fat and nonfat choices. Be aware, however, that the law of averages does not permit you to eat an unlimited amount of foods that are 20 percent fat or higher. If you do that, you'll tip the balance beyond the point where nonfat or low-fat foods can bring you back to the middle.

The following guidelines will help you use the law of averages to reach your 10 percent goal:

- Choose as many foods as possible that are free of fat or nearly nonfat.

- Cut back drastically on foods that get more than 20 percent of their calories from fat.

- Eat thoughtfully and carefully those foods which get between 10 and 20 percent of their calories from fat.

Counting fat grams: Another approach for controlling your fat intake is to count fat grams. This method may seem laborious at first, but once you are familiar with the number of fat grams in each portion of the foods you usually eat, the process becomes very simple, and it will give you an accurate picture of how much fat you're eating.

To begin, use the following tables to find your personal daily fat-gram target. This number will represent the maximum amount of fat grams that a person of your sex, activity level, and desirable weight can consume each day without exceeding the 10 percent guideline. Here's what to do:

CHART 1: DESIRABLE WEIGHTS[1] FOR MEN (Ages 25 And Over)

Height[2]				
Feet	Inches	Small Frame	Medium Frame	Large Frame
5	2	112-120	118-129	126-141
5	3	115-123	121-133	129-144
5	4	118-126	124-136	132-148
5	5	121-129	127-139	135-152
5	6	124-133	130-143	138-156
5	7	128-137	134-147	142-161
5	8	132-141	138-152	147-166
5	9	136-145	142-156	151-170
5	10	140-150	146-160	155-174
5	11	144-154	150-165	159-179
6	0	148-158	154-170	164-184
6	1	152-162	158-175	168-189
6	2	156-167	162-180	173-194
6	3	160-171	167-185	178-199
6	4	164-175	172-190	182-204

[1]*Weight in pounds according to frame (indoor clothing).*
[2]*With 1-inch heel shoes on.*

SOURCE: *Metropolitan Life Insurance Company Actuarial Tables, 1959.*

To determine your ideal weight, find your height in the left-hand column. Then move across the page to the body frame that best describes you. For the purposes of this table, your body frame is "small" if you can wrap your left thumb and middle finger around your right wrist and have these two digits overlap. If the thumb and finger barely touch, then you have a "medium" body frame. If they don't touch at all, you have a "large" build.

1. Use the charts on this or the next page to find the desirable weight for your sex and height. The weight on these charts will tell you how much you should be for your height and bone structure—not necessarily how much you actually weigh. If you are overweight now, the foods you select under this program are likely to help you lose weight.

(While these charts from the Metropolitan Life Insurance Company can give you a sense of whether you are overweight, a more accurate indicator is to have your body fat percentage calculated—with skin-fold measurements, for example, or underwater weighing—which is a better reflection of your ideal weight and health status than your absolute weight. Men should try to maintain their body fat at no more than 20 percent; women should aim for under 30 percent—the closer to 25 percent, the better.)

CHART 2: DESIRABLE WEIGHTS[1] FOR WOMEN (Ages 25 And Over)

Height[2]		Small Frame	Medium Frame	Large Frame
Feet	Inches			
4	10	92-98	96-107	104-119
4	11	94-101	98-110	106-122
5	0	96-104	101-113	109-125
5	1	99-107	104-116	112-128
5	2	102-110	107-119	115-131
5	3	105-113	110-122	118-134
5	4	108-116	113-126	121-138
5	5	111-119	116-130	125-142
5	6	114-123	120-135	129-146
5	7	118-127	124-139	133-150
5	8	122-131	128-143	137-154
5	9	126-135	132-147	141-158
5	10	130-140	136-151	145-163
5	11	134-144	140-155	149-168
6	0	138-148	144-159	153-173

[1]*Weight in pounds according to frame (indoor clothing).*
[2]*With 2-inch heel shoes on.*

SOURCE: *Metropolitan Life Insurance Company Actuarial Tables,* 1959.

2. Next, determine your general physical activity level:

Inactive: You fall into this category if your physical activity is limited. Perhaps you do some occasional slow walking. Or you may concentrate on recreational activities such as fishing, golf (with the help of a golf cart), bowling, or horseback riding.

Moderately Active: In this category, your activities would include ten to twenty minutes a day of continuous vigorous exercise, three or more times a week. These activities could range from jogging to swimming to skiing to doubles tennis.

Active: You belong in this category if you spend over twenty minutes exercising continuously and vigorously, three or more times a week. These activities might include jogging, swimming, singles tennis, or full court basketball. (Even if you're not at this level now, you may be soon by incorporating the exercise components of this program into your lifestyle.)

3.   Finally, with your ideal weight and activity level in mind, consult the charts on the next two pages to determine your own fat-gram number. You will use this number to help

CHART 3: PERSONAL DAILY FAT-GRAM TARGETS: MEN

Desirable Weight	Activity Level		
	Inactive	Moderately Active	Very Active
90	14	15	16
100	16	17	18
110	17	18	20
120	19	20	21
130	20	22	23
140	22	23	25
150	23	25	27
160	25	27	28
170	26	28	30
180	28	30	32
190	30	32	34
200	31	33	36
210	33	35	37
220	34	37	39

Find the figure in the left-hand column that most closely corresponds to the desirable weight you identified in Step 1. Then move across the chart to the vertical column that corresponds to your physical activity level. At the point where your ideal weight and activity level intersect, you will find your personal fat-gram number. This number represents the maximum amount of fat (in grams) that you should consume each day.

you channel your eating behavior in a more positive direction. Follow the instructions that appear beneath the chart.

Let's say, for example, that you're a woman with a desirable weight of 130 pounds, and you're moderately active. Move across and down the appropriate columns in Chart 4, and you'll find that your personal fat-gram number is 20—that is, you should try to limit the amount of total fat you consume each day to 20 grams.

You will use your fat-gram number to guide you in your food selections and meal planning, and to keep track of how much fat you're consuming during the day. Write down everything you eat, and next to each food item, the grams of fat in that food.

CHART 4: PERSONAL DAILY FAT-GRAM TARGETS: WOMEN

	Activity Level		
Desirable Weight	**Inactive**	**Moderately Active**	**Very Active**
90	13	14	14
100	14	15	16
110	15	17	18
120	17	18	19
130	18	20	21
140	20	21	22
150	21	23	24
160	22	24	26
170	24	26	27
180	25	27	29
190	27	29	30
200	28	30	32
210	29	32	34
220	31	33	35

Find the figure in the left-hand column that most closely corresponds to the desirable weight you identified in Step 1. Then move across the chart to the vertical column that corresponds to your physical activity level. At the point where your ideal weight and activity level intersect, you will find your personal fat-gram number. This number represents the maximum amount of fat (in grams) that you should consume each day.

How can you determine just how many fat grams a particular food has? Or if you're using the "law of averages" technique, how can you find out the percentage of calories from fat in the foods you eat?

Later in this section, you will find some examples of common foods, with values for both their total fat grams in a typical serving and their percentage of fat calories. We also suggest that you purchase a "fat counter" booklet, which will give you this same information on every conceivable food item—many more foods than we could ever publish in this book. Another excellent source of fat figures is food labels themselves, which appear on all packaged food.

MAKING THE BEST USE OF FOOD LABELS

In 1994, the Food and Drug Administration began requiring food manufacturers to display new nutritional labels on most foods. These "Nutritional Facts" labels make the fat content of foods and other information very accessible.

The most important items on the food label for our program are: *Serving Size, Calories, Calories from Fat,* and *Total Fat.*

Serving Size. Most of us have our own idea of what constitutes a "serving." For some people, a serving of chicken means a boneless breast; for others, it's a breast, a thigh, a wing, and a leg. For some, a serving of pasta is just enough to cover a small plate; for others, it's a pile of spaghetti four inches high that spans a large dish.

Unfortunately, our ideas about serving size rarely match up with the ones that food manufacturers list on nutritional labels. In most cases, our servings are much more generous. Pasta is one of the best examples of this discrepancy. Although the manufacturer insists there are eight servings in each box of spaghetti, my wife and I routinely cook half the box for the two of us. Bagels are another good example. Did you know that one bagel is considered two servings?

Manufacturers are purposely stingy with their portion sizes to make it look like you're getting more for your money. You might not buy a $4 box of breakfast cereal that says it contains only four servings. When the box claims to contain ten, it seems like a bargain. Decreasing the serving size also makes the product look more appealing from a nutritional standpoint. A smaller serving size automatically contains less fat than a larger one.

Regardless of what the label says, your serving size is the amount you choose to put on your plate. So, even if you are selecting low-fat or nonfat foods, you can totally undermine your efforts by overloading on them. Pretzels are a good example. Pretzels are considered a low-fat snack, because most pretzels get only 10 to 20 percent of their calories from fat. One ounce of almost any pretzel (that's the official serving size) contains 2 grams of fat and 110 calories. But who eats just one ounce? The average person would consider two or three ounces a "normal" serving—still a relatively small amount of food, but between 4 and 6 fat grams and 220 and 330 calories worth of energy. That number of fat grams may be more than you bargained for in a low-fat snack.

Nutrition Facts	
Serving Size ½ cup (114g)	
Servings Per Container 4	

Amount Per Serving	
Calories 90	Calories from Fat 30

	% Daily Value*
Total Fat 3g	**5%**
Saturated Fat 0g	0%
Cholesterol 0mg	**0%**
Sodium 300mg	**13%**
Total Carbohydrate 13g	**4%**
Dietary Fiber 3g	12%
Sugars 3g	
Protein 3g	

Vitamin A	80%	Vitamin C	60%
Calcium	4%	Iron	4%

* Percent Daily Values are based on a 2,000 calorie diet. Your daily values may be higher or lower depending on your calorie needs:

		Calories	2,000	2,500
Total Fat	Less than		65g	80g
Sat Fat	Less than		20g	25g
Cholesterol	Less than		300mg	300mg
Sodium	Less than		2,400mg	2,400mg
Total Carbohydrate			300g	375g
Fiber			25g	30g

Calories per gram:
Fat 9   •   Carbohydrate 4   •   Protein 4

So, what's my advice? Read labels before you buy any food, and take a careful look at the manufacturer's portion size. Don't let yourself be tricked into buying foods that will end up stuffing you with more fat grams than you expected.

Calories. Although calories aren't as important to this fitness program as fat, it's very useful to know the number of calories contained in the given serving size, particularly if you're trying to lose weight. Generally, you're better off selecting foods that have a low number of calories and a large serving size; they'll be low in fat as well.

Calories from Fat. These calories indicate the actual number of fat calories in each serving size. This figure includes all types of fat (saturated, monounsaturated, polyunsaturated).

You can use the numbers listed for *Calories* and *Calories from Fat* to determine the percentage of calories from fat in a given serving. This information is crucial if you're using the law of averages to keep your fat intake at about 10 percent of calories. Here's how to make this calculation:

- Divide the number of *Calories from Fat* by the total *Calories* in the serving size.

- Take the result, and multiply it by 100 to change it to a percentage. (The fastest way to change the result into a percentage is to move the decimal point two digits to the right.) This figure is the *percentage of calories that comes from fat.*

THE NEW FOOD-LABEL TERMINOLOGY

Federal regulations have standardized the meaning of key words that often appear on food packaging. The FDA has prescribed the definitions listed here for the following terms:

Fat-Free: Less than 0.5 grams of fat per serving. You should increase most dramatically these foods in your diet.

Low-Fat: Three grams or less of fat per serving. You can occasionally eat these foods without concern, unless you eat several servings.

Lean: Less than ten grams of fat, four grams of saturated fat, and 95 milligrams of cholesterol per serving. You need to be careful with these foods and read the rest of the label carefully, since they can contain as many as 89 fat calories per serving.

Light (Lite): One-third fewer calories, or no more than one-half the fat of the higher-calorie, higher-fat version. These foods are potentially risky; if you're consuming "light" granola that has one-half the fat of the higher-fat granola, you'll still be eating lots of fat.

Cholesterol-Free: Less than two milligrams of cholesterol and two grams (or less) of saturated fat per serving. The risk here is that the food contains lots of unsaturated fat (perhaps vegetable oils), which will contribute to your overall fat intake.

For example, using the sample label on page 24, you would divide 30 (the number of *Calories from Fat*) by 90 (the number of *Calories* in a serving), arriving at a result of .33.

Then multiply that figure by 100, converting it to 33 percent. In this example, this particular food would not be encouraged on our program (or it would have to be eaten *very* sparingly) because of the high percentage of its calories that comes from fat.

Total Fat (in grams). If you're counting fat grams as your way of monitoring your fat intake, the lower the *Total Fat* content on the label, the better. In the sample label, the *Total Fat* for this item is 3 grams per serving; you count this number if you decide to eat this food. Remember, however, if you consume more than the serving size listed—let's say 1 cup rather than the 1/2 cup listed on the label—you'd have to adjust your intake of *Total Fat* grams accordingly (in our example, doubling it from 3 grams to 6).

CHOOSING FOOD ON THIS PROGRAM

In this plan, you need to avoid or drastically minimize your consumption of all foods that derive more than 20 percent of their calories from fat. By reading food labels carefully, and using a food-counter book as well, you'll discover for yourself the foods that do and don't belong in your supermarket shopping cart.

Meat and Fish

You do not need to eliminate meat from your diet completely. Because most meat is high in total fat, you should cut back on the amount you consume. Choose the cuts that are lowest in fat, and limit portion sizes. Neither of these actions is as difficult as you may think.

In recent years, meat producers have adopted new breeding and feeding methods that have reduced the fat content of their animals. Even so, beef is still a major source of fat in the American diet. In general, you should eat beef less frequently, and even then only with care. When choosing beef, concentrate on cuts that have the least amount of visible fat or marbling throughout the muscle. Also keep in mind that even when beef appears lean, it still has lots of fat. As the table *Fat Content of Common Meat and Fish* on the next page shows, cuts such as eye of round and top round have less fat than other cuts, containing 20 percent or less of fat calories. Avoid the fattiest cuts, which include ribs and tenderloin. Look for low-fat grades of ground beef, too. And stay away from liver, kidney, heart, and tongue, except on rare occasions.

Keep your portion sizes small as well. I recommend about three or four ounces per serving. That's a piece approximately the size of a deck of playing cards. You can further cut the amount of fat in each serving of meat by extending these dishes with beans, pastas, grains, and vegetables that are low in fat. Try adding rice, barley, potatoes, or carrots to a meat recipe; you won't lose much of the robust meat flavor that you may enjoy, but you will lose some of meat's potential to add pounds to your waistline.

In many (though certainly not all) instances, you are better off choosing poultry or fish than beef. Depending on the type you choose, poultry or fish can be lower in total fat. For instance, in seafood, fat levels are especially low in cod, haddock, and yellowfin tuna. Types of seafood that are higher in fat include bass, herring, and sardines. Cooked freshwater bass, for instance, contains four grams of total fat in a three-ounce serving, so that about 29 percent of its calories come from fat. Compare those numbers to those for the same size serving of haddock, which contains less than one gram of fat and gets about 8 percent of its calories from fat.

When choosing chicken and turkey, bear in mind that light meat contains less fat than dark meat. If you choose dark meat, you may not be any better off than you would be if you ate beef. While skinless dark chicken meat contains 8.3 grams of total fat in a typical three-ounce cooked serving (43 percent of calories from fat), skinless white meat (breast) contains much less: 3.1 grams (20 percent of calories from fat). Removing the skin before eating can make a big difference in the fat content; if you leave the skin on that serving of light chicken meat, the percentage of calories from fat nearly doubles.

One other note about poultry: Ground chicken or turkey may not be as low in fat as you

FAT CONTENT OF COMMON MEAT AND FISH

	Portion	Total Fat (grams)	% Fat Calories
Bass, freshwater, broiled	3 oz.	4.0	29%
Beef, eye of round, lean, trimmed, roasted	3 oz.	3.0	20%
Beef rib, small end, lean, trimmed, broiled	3 oz.	7.4	40%
Beef tenderloin, lean, trimmed, broiled	3 oz.	7.5	40%
Beef, tip round, lean, trimmed, roasted	3 oz.	4.5	28%
Beef, top round, lean, trimmed, braised	3 oz.	3.4	19%
Beef, top sirloin, lean, trimmed, broiled	3 oz.	4.8	28%
Chicken breast, with skin, roasted	3 oz.	6.6	36%
Chicken breast, without skin, roasted	3 oz.	3.1	20%
Chicken, dark meat, without skin, roasted	3 oz.	8.3	43%
Cod, Atlantic, broiled	3 oz.	0.7	7%
Ground beef, 7% fat by weight, broiled or baked	3 oz.	7.0	42%
Haddock, broiled	3 oz.	0.8	8%
Halibut, broiled	3 oz.	2.5	19%
Salmon, pink, broiled	3 oz.	3.8	27%
Tuna, yellowfin, fresh, broiled	3 oz.	1.0	8%
Turkey, dark meat, without skin, roasted	3 oz.	6.1	35%
Turkey, light meat, without skin, roasted	3 oz.	2.7	18%

think, unless you have it ground to order. Manufacturers of commercially ground poultry are permitted to grind some skin in with the rest of the chicken or turkey, significantly raising the percentage of calories from fat. You might consider grinding skinless turkey breast in your own meat grinder so that you keep the fat content right where it belongs.

Dairy Products

Dairy products are important and economical sources of calcium, protein, and vitamin D. However, if you don't select the right products, this food category can also become a very troublesome source of excess fat. For example, you need to choose cheese carefully and eat it in smaller amounts than you may be used to.

Although whole milk and low-fat milk are 3.3 percent and 2 percent fat respectively by weight, those numbers are actually quite misleading, because milk is mostly water. When you calculate the actual number of calories in milk that comes from fat, the figures are unsettling. In whole milk (total calories: 150 per eight-ounce glass), 49 percent of the calories are fat calories; that figure drops (but not by much) to 37 percent for 2 percent milk (total calories: 121 per glass). You're much better off choosing "nonfat" or skim milk, which gets only about 4 percent of its calories from fat (total calories: 86 per glass).

FAT CONTENT OF COMMON DAIRY PRODUCTS

	Portion	Total Fat (grams)	% Fat Calories
American cheese, fat-free singles	1 oz.	0	0%
Butter	1 tbs. or 3 pats	12.2	100%
Cheddar cheese, mild or sharp	1 oz.	2.0	36%
Cottage cheese, 1% fat	.5 cup	1.2	13%
Cottage cheese, 2% fat	.5 cup	2.2	20%
Cream, coffee	1 tbs.	2.9	90%
Milk, evaporated, skim, canned	.5 cup	0.3	3%
Milk, skim or nonfat	1 cup	0.4	4%
Milk, 1% fat	1 cup	2.6	23%
Milk, 2% fat	1 cup	5.0	37%
Milk, whole	1 cup	8.2	49%
Mozzarella cheese, reduced-fat	1 oz.	3.0	39%
Mozzarella cheese, fat-free	1 oz.	0	0%
Ricotta cheese, part-skim	1 oz.	2.2	51%
Sour cream, reduced-fat	1 oz.	3.0	68%
Swiss cheese	1 oz.	7.8	66%
Yogurt, 1% milkfat, fruit on bottom	8 oz.	3.0	11%
Yogurt, nonfat, vanilla	8 oz.	0	0%

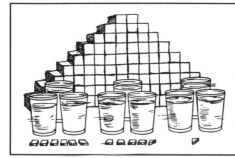

Making the switch from whole milk to nonfat milk can significantly reduce your fat intake. If you were to drink three glasses of whole milk a day for a year, you'd consume fat equal to the amount in 88 sticks of butter. On a daily basis, drinking three glasses of whole milk would be equivalent to consuming six pats of butter, compared to 4-1/2 pats with low-fat milk and 1/2 pat with nonfat.

Cheese tends to be brimming with fat; in most cheeses, 65 to 75 percent of the calories comes from fat. Even the "low-fat" or "part-skim" cheeses contain more than you might think. For example, part-skim ricotta, although lower in fat than the whole milk variety, still has a fat content equal to 51 percent of its calories. Some "fat-free" varieties of cheese are now available, and although their flavor and texture may not be as good as the real thing, many people have adapted well to them, and use them in salads and sauces.

Since you can choose so many other dairy foods that are low in fat, and since most cheeses (except the fat-free varieties) are way over our 30 percent fat guideline, if you love cheese, I suggest treating it as a delicacy. That means eating cheese less often and in much smaller portions, and trying to stick with the low-fat or nonfat alternatives. Limit your portion sizes to about one-third of what you would have eaten in the past. Another way to beat the fat trap is to grate Parmesan, cheddar, or sapsago cheese, and sprinkle it on casseroles or main dishes; you'll be able to enjoy the flavor of cheese without sabotaging your fat-lowering efforts.

Many lower-fat dairy alternatives are now available in your supermarket, including fat-free frozen dairy desserts and nonfat yogurt, which can be used as a substitute for sour cream in recipes (A cup of plain nonfat yogurt has no fat, while an equal amount of regular sour cream contains about 42 grams!) You can also eliminate a lot of fat by using nonfat yogurt as a salad dressing or as a topping for baked potatoes. As for butter and margarine, they will cost you dearly in terms of fat content. All of butter's calories come from fat. And don't expect to fare any better with margarine, because 100 percent of its calories are derived from fat, too.

You can cut back on the fat a little by selecting reduced-calorie or diet varieties of margarine. Since they are diluted with water, tablespoon for tablespoon they have as little as half the fat (and half the calories) of regular margarine. But their percentage of fat is still far above the 20 percent limit we've established for most foods in this eating plan, so you really ought to use jam or jelly on your morning toast instead. If you can't bear the thought of giving up butter or margarine completely, save it for special occasions, and then cut your portion size to one-third of what you once used. You'll still get the feel and flavor, but without all the extra fat. (See *Fat Content of Common Dairy Products*, on the previous page.)

Oils

When heart disease is the concern, some oils (monounsaturated, polyunsaturated) are better than others. When overall fitness is your goal, however, all oils should be treated identically—by avoiding or drastically reducing your intake of them. They are all 100 percent fat.

Food manufacturers are making it very easy to cut back on fat from one source: salad dressings. Fat-free dressings have become widely available, and contain no fat, no cholesterol, and relatively few calories. If you are using a higher-fat dressing, however, in which more than 30 percent of calories come from fat, you need to use much less of it—about one-third of what you once used.

FAT CONTENT OF COMMON OILS AND SPREADS

	Portion	Total Fat (grams)	% Fat Calories
Canola oil	1 tbs.	13.6	100%
Margarine, regular, soft	1 tbs.	11.0	100%
Margarine, whipped	1 tbs.	7.0	90%
Margarine, soft, reduced-calorie	1 tbs.	6.0	84%
Margarine, soft, extra-light spread, tub	1 tbs.	4.0	80%
Mayonnaise, cholesterol-free, reduced-calorie	1 tbs.	5.0	90%
Mayonnaise, dressing, nonfat	1 tbs.	0	0%
Olive oil	1 tbs.	13.5	100%
Safflower oil	1 tbs.	13.6	100%

Snacks And Desserts

As with salad dressings, snacks and desserts need not undermine your low-fat dietary program. Your supermarket carries dozens of low-fat and nonfat snack foods and desserts; even some cookies and cakes qualify. Some premium ice creams now come in fat-free

HEART SMART VERSUS DIET SMART

The fats we are most concerned with in this program come in three types: saturated, polyunsaturated, and monounsaturated fatty acids. These fatty acids differ from one another in their chemical structure. Most foods that contain fat have all three types, but in varying proportions. Depending on which type of fat predominates in a particular food, the food is considered to be saturated, polyunsaturated, or monounsaturated.

Saturated fats are the biggest contributor to heart disease. But when your goal is overall fitness, you need to cut back on your intake of all three types of fat. All three kinds are 100 percent fat, and add to your total fat intake.

varieties, containing zero fat and zero cholesterol in flavors as irresistible as chocolate fudge. Most commercial ice cream and yogurt shops now offer nonfat versions of their desserts, too, but you still need to be careful with your portion sizes.

Let's not forget about the wonderful desserts and snacks that nature created for us. Frankly, if you're looking for a very low-fat treat, you can't do any better than to select a tasty fruit. Or you can air-pop some popcorn, sprinkling it with a little Parmesan cheese or herbs or spices for flavor. (See *Fat Content of Common Snacks and Desserts* below.)

FAT CONTENT OF COMMON SNACKS AND DESSERTS

	Portion	Total Fat (grams)	% Fat Calories
Applesauce, unsweetened	.5 cup	0.1	2%
Dairy dessert, nonfat	.5 cup	0	0%
Popcorn, microwavable, light, butter-flavored	3 cups	2.0	30%
Popcorn, popped without fat, salted	3 cups	1.2	12%
Sherbet	.5 cup	1.0	8%
Strawberries, fresh	.5 cup	0.3	12%
Yogurt, frozen, low-fat	3 fluid oz.	1.0	7%
Yogurt, frozen, nonfat	3 fluid oz.	0	0%

Other Low-Fat Choices

In the 2000 revision of the federal government's *Dietary Guidelines for Americans*, the report advised using grains, vegetables and fruits as the foundation of a good diet. Meats, poultry and dairy products were relegated to a smaller role and Americans were urged to "go easy" on foods high in fat and sugars. Also, for the first time in 1996, the expert panel noted that vegetarianism is a health-promoting way of eating, although individuals who avoid animal products must be sure to get enough iron, vitamin B_{12}, calcium, and zinc in their diets.

As you've read in the preceding pages, however, you don't have to give up meat or dairy products to succeed with this program. Even so, the vegetarian's reliance on lots of fruits, vegetables, legumes, grains and cereals is how you should be thinking. As you cut back on meat, replace it with these low-fat alternatives. When you fill up your plate with vegetables—as long as they're prepared without butter, fatty dressings, or sauces—you'll be on your way to a diet containing 10 percent fat. Eat plenty of brown rice, beans, breads and cereals, too, and you will succeed in reaching your low-fat goals. See the sections on *Cholesterol* (pages 95-113) and *Fiber* (pages 137-139) for more information on making healthy foods part of your diet.

THE RISK OF HIGH-PROTEIN DIETS

If weight loss is one of your goals, an array of high-protein (and often high-fat) diets have probably caught your attention in recent years. The Atkins and the Zone diets are probably the best known of these programs, but there are many others—including the Sugar Busters and Stillman diets—that have also gained popularity, but have come under the scrutiny of the American Heart Association (AHA).

While it's true that you may be able to lose weight *over the short term* on high protein diets, largely through the diuretic effect of reductions in carbohydrate intake, the AHA became so concerned about the high-protein programs that it issued an advisory in its medical journal, *Circulation*, in 2001. This report noted that a high-protein diet has no proven effectiveness in long-term weight management, while also posing health threats over the long term.

According to the AHA statement, as these diets increase protein and fat intake, many also reduce the consumption of fruits, vegetables and other nutritionally beneficial foods. They can fall short in providing adequate vitamins, minerals and fiber. The high-protein regimens may also pose particular risks for people with liver and kidney disease in whom excess protein could exacerbate their diseases.

While people do need protein in their diet for good health, most Americans already consume more protein than their bodies require. So with weight loss in mind, here's what I suggest: Minimize your caloric intake, while also ensuring that you're eating a balanced diet that includes plenty of grains, fruits, and vegetables, as well as some protein.

Vegetarian Diets: Not A Low-Fat Guarantee

Many vegetarians assume—incorrectly—that a meat-free diet translates into a low-fat diet. After all, vegetables are generally low in fat, right? Right, but vegetarians do not live on vegetables alone. Although some very strict vegetarians avoid dairy products, most rely quite heavily on them as a source of protein, which can cause problems with fat intake. For example, many vegetarians substitute cheese for meat, chicken, and fish, yet many cheeses derive more than 60 percent of their calories from fat (by comparison, skinless breast of chicken derives only 20 percent of its calories from fat, and cod only 7 percent).

Oils present another problem. Many vegetarian recipes call for lots of added fat in the form of oils, butter, or margarine. This extra fat is used to enhance the flavor of the low-fat vegetables, legumes, and grains that are the staples of many vegetarian dishes.

Unfortunately, flavor is not the only thing added. Every tablespoon of oil adds 120 calories to the dish—100 percent of them fat calories.

And then there's the problem of snack foods and desserts. High-fat cakes and cookies don't lose their fat when they're eaten by vegetarians.

So, if you're a vegetarian, don't assume you are automatically on a low-fat diet. Give as much thought to the percentage of fat in the foods you choose to eat as you do in any other diet.

SOME FINAL TIPS

Because of the enormous health benefits associated with low-fat eating, why doesn't everyone keep a lid on his or her fat consumption? Some people truly believe that a life with little fat is a life with little joy. They love the taste and the feel of fat—its moisture and its smooth texture on the tongue and the palate. Many of the foods they've grown up with are high in fat, and they simply aren't used to cooking and eating any other way. In short, they find the richness of fat too appetizing and palatable to forsake.

But they haven't discovered just how pleasurable low-fat dining can be. Here are some final suggestions you can use to make your meals both low-fat and delectable:

- Avoid frying (which increases the food's fat content because it literally adds fat to the basic food), relying instead on methods that permit the fat to drip off during cooking—including broiling, baking, roasting, and braising. Also, remember that medium or well-done meat will tend to have less fat than rare meat, since fat continues to be lost as long as the cooking process continues. Be sure you have trimmed away all visible fat before cooking. Since lean beef cooks faster than fattier cuts, cook it for about 20 percent less time than you would cook beef that is higher in fat. Beef that is overcooked will probably be tougher than you'd like.

- Use nonstick cookware. Instead of cooking with butter, use a little nonstick cooking spray.

- Refrigerate soups, stews, and sauces before serving them. When you take them out of the refrigerator, the fat will have congealed at the top. Skim it off the surface before reheating.

- For pancake and waffle toppings, use fresh fruit (strawberries, blueberries) or applesauce. Fruit can also be added to many muffin and pancake recipes.

- Begin cooking with half the amount of fat called for in the recipe. In general, you won't need to add any more, and the chemistry of the recipe won't be significantly altered. Vegetables with strong aromas (onions, peppers, celery, garlic) can enhance the flavor of many dishes with substantially reduced fat content.

- Use some creativity in making low-fat substitutions when preparing food. For instance, instead of putting butter on your baked potato, try salsa. Rather than cooking with whole-milk cheddar cheese, use part-skim mozzarella.

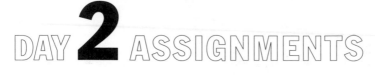

DAY **2** ASSIGNMENTS

MET GOAL   PARTIALLY MET GOAL   MISSED GOAL

PHYSICAL VITALITY

1. Improve your time for the measured mile by 2 seconds.   **Time:**_____
2. Do all the flexibility and stretching exercises.

NUTRITIONAL VITALITY

3. Decrease total fat intake to 10% of total calories.
4. Eat at least 7 half-cup portions of fruits and vegetables.

MENTAL VITALITY

EMOTIONAL & SPIRITUAL VITALITY

MEDICAL VITALITY

IMPROVING
YOUR FLEXIBILITY   DAY 2

In the physical side of our vitality program, you'll find key elements that include aerobic activity and strength training. But now it's time to start working on the first element: flexibility. For the average person, flexibility is just as important as the other two physical parts of our program, because it helps prevent many of the common aches and pains of daily living. Joints that are flexible will move freely and comfortably through the full range of motion for which they are "designed." Inflexible joints interfere with the body's ability to perform simple movements and are a common cause of pain.

Maintaining your flexibility can make a big difference in your daily life. A limber neck allows you to look backward without discomfort; a flexible shoulder lets you screw in a light bulb overhead without fear of pain. Being flexible also protects you against muscle injury if the intensity of your other exercise activities reaches high levels.

Some people appear to be generally more or less flexible than others. These differences are probably due to hereditary factors. However, in the same way that strength is specific to each muscle, flexibility is specific to each joint of the body. Therefore, some joints in the body may be quite inflexible when compared with other joints. Fortunately, the flexibility of any healthy joint can be improved with stretching exercises, which you'll find in this chapter.

Most people believe that they will lose flexibility as they grow older, because inflexibility is so common among older people. But this loss is the result of inactivity, not the natural consequence of aging. Muscles that are not stretched become shorter, and joints that are not moved become stiffer and painful. Before long, it becomes too painful to move the joints through their full range, so their motion is restricted even further. A vicious cycle of declining use and declining function follows. This problem can almost always be prevented with regular stretching exercises.

PROMOTING FLEXIBILITY

Each element in our program has its own unique process for development. To develop aerobic fitness, you must exercise vigorously enough to raise your heart rate for sustained periods of time. To build strength, you must work your muscles against increasing levels of resistance. To promote flexibility, you need to stretch the muscles and connective tissues that bind to your joints.

Stretching exercises extend muscles just a little beyond their current length, which in most people is less than what they could be. With time, however, these regularly stretched muscles adjust to a new length and elasticity, improving the range of motion of the joint.

Try this brief set of simple motions, which will give you a sense of just how flexible you are now:

1. Bring your chin down to your chest. Can you put your chin on your chest without feeling any discomfort in your neck? Note how close you can get before any pain starts.

2. Turn your head as far to the right as it will go. Now to the left. How far behind yourself can you see without discomfort or pain? Note your position and the farthest point you can see without causing discomfort, so you can repeat this test again.

3. Stand up with your arms dangling at your sides, with palms facing inwards. Raise your right arm to the side through a full half-circle until your hand is as high over your head as you can comfortably reach. Repeat with your left arm. Note the highest position you can reach without causing pain or discomfort in your shoulder.

4. With your legs straight and your hands outstretched above your head, slowly bend at the waist until your hands are pointing toward your toes. Do not force your hands toward your toes; instead, simply let the weight of your upper body lower your hands as close as they will go to the floor. How many inches away from the floor are the tips of your fingers? (To measure this distance easily, place a tall stack of books on the floor and slide books off the stack with your outstretched fingertips until you can't reach the next book. Then measure the height of the stack to determine the distance of your fingertips from the floor. Or lean a 12-inch ruler against the wall, and use it as your measuring instrument.)

Keep track of your performance on each of these simple flexibility tests. During the coming weeks, you should repeat these tests to see how much you've been able to increase your flexibility with the simple stretching exercises you'll find in this program.

HOW TO STRETCH PROPERLY

Each stretching session should begin with a simple warm-up routine. A warm-up routine reduces the risk of discomfort or injury. Spend five to ten minutes doing any light exercise—slow walking, "jogging" in place, or gently pedaling an exercise cycle, for example, to warm up your muscles. Then you are ready to start stretching.

The safest way to stretch a muscle is to apply a sustained "static" stretch, keeping the muscle relaxed and motionless while it is being stretched. We now know that a once-popular stretching technique, "ballistic stretching," can actually be harmful. This technique uses "bobbing" or "bouncing" movements to force the stretch. Unfortunately, these motions cause the muscle to contract and stretch at the same time. This combination can produce soreness and damage to the muscle.

There are actually two parts to "the stretch." In the first part you are merely extending yourself to the *natural* limit of your body's movement *at that time*. It's a limit you can improve upon with stretching exercises.

Then, in the second part of the stretch, move just a little beyond your natural limit until you reach a point where you can feel the stretch. You shouldn't feel pain, but you will feel tension forming within your tissues. This position will give you increased flexibility and new limits. It is a position of growth.

The difference between your first and final positions might be no more than 1/8 to 1/4 inch, but there may be a great difference in the way they feel to you. Neither position should ever feel painful. If it does, you're stretching too far. As you progress, you will be starting many sessions at a point more flexible than the initial position of your prior session.

Before you start, here are a couple of tips to make stretching work better for you:

1. Always do your stretching slowly and steadily. Rapid, jerky motions may cause you to stretch too far, resulting in discomfort or injury. As you do your stretching exercises, you should simply stretch until you feel tightness in your tissues. Hold this position. If those tissues *hurt*, the pain is your signal to back off. When you're stretching one part of your body, try to keep all the other parts relaxed. Take slow, deep breaths. Concentrate on nothing but the part being stretched

2. Unless indicated differently in the exercises below, hold each stretch for at least six seconds, preferably as much as 20 seconds or even more.

THE STRETCHING PROGRAM

Here is the program you can start today. These exercises were chosen because they're safe, no matter what your particular level of fitness is. As you perform them over the next few weeks, take note of the increasing flexibility you will be gaining. At the end of this program, you'll find several ideas for extending your stretching program to all parts of your body. Set aside 5 to 10 minutes to warm up, and then another 10 to 15 minutes for the exercises themselves.

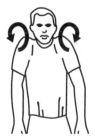
Slowly circle shoulders backward 8-12 times. Repeat, circling shoulders forward 8-12 times.

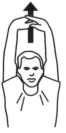
Interlock your fingers above your head. Push your arms slightly back and up. Hold the stretch 15-30 seconds. Repeat 2-3 times.

Illustrations ©Willis-Knighton Fitness and Wellness Centers; used with permission.

Stand with your feet about shoulder width apart and toes pointed straight ahead. Keeping your knees slightly bent, reach overhead with one arm, with the other arm down by the side. Slowly lean to the side at your waist until you feel a good stretch. Hold this position 15-30 seconds. Repeat on the other side.

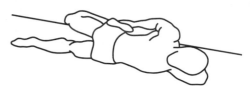

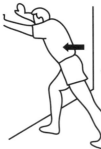

Stand facing the wall with one foot approximately 2 feet in front of the other. Slowly bend the front knee until you feel mild tension in the back calf muscle. Hold this position 15-30 seconds. Keep your toes pointed straight ahead and your heels on the ground. Repeat with the other leg.

Hold your right foot with your right hand and gently pull the heel toward your body. Hold the stretch for 15-30 seconds once you feel tension in the quadriceps muscle. Repeat on the other leg.

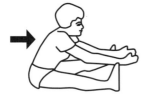

Sit with your legs at a comfortable distance apart and your back straight. Reach forward with the arms, bending at the hips until you feel a slight tension in the groin area. Hold 15-30 seconds. Repeat 2-3 times.

Stand on one leg with the other propped on a support. Slowly bend forward from the hips keeping the back straight until you feel a stretch in your hamstring. Hold this position 15-30 seconds. Repeat with the other leg.

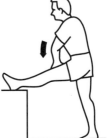

Lie on your back. Bend one knee, placing your foot on the floor. Grasp the straight leg and slowly pull your leg toward your body until you feel tension in the hamstring. Hold this position 15-30 seconds. Repeat with the other leg.

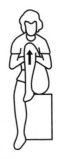

Sit on a chair with your back straight. Lift one leg and bend the knee. Hold behind the knee and slowly pull the leg toward the body until you feel a stretch in the hamstring. Hold this position 15-30 seconds. Repeat with the other leg.

As you perform these stretching exercises, day after day, you will enjoy the way your body is changing as your flexibility and range of motion improve. Concentrate not just on how the muscles and tissues feel as they're being stretched, but also on how they feel when the stretch is over. You'll see how relaxed they become—and how good you feel—as they return to their more natural state. You'll also find that as your flexibility increases, some of your aches and pains may disappear.

Keep in mind that this chapter is only an introduction to flexibility. If you'd like to expand your own flexibility program, including incorporating more exercises into it, here are some books we recommend:

- *Stretching* by Bob Anderson (Shelter Publications)
- *Stretching at Your Computer or Desk* by Bob Anderson (Shelter Publications)
- *Sports Stretching* by Michael J. Alter (Human Kinetics)

MUSCLE STRETCHING DO'S AND DON'TS

Do's

1. Always do a general warm-up routine before you start stretching any individual muscles.
2. Hold stretches at least six seconds, up to 20 or more seconds. This will ensure that the maximum benefit of stretching takes place.
3. Stretch only to the point of tightness, not to the point of pain.
4. Relax and breathe deeply while stretching.
5. Move slowly into and out of each stretch.
6. Stretch often, if possible every day, and even multiple times per day.

Don'ts

1. Do not bounce during stretches.
2. Do not perform the following stretches:

    (a) Stretching the neck backwards. (This can interfere with blood flow to the head.)

    (b) Hyperextending, or locking, the knee. (This is an unnatural position for the knee and can weaken the joint.)

    (c) "Plow" or raise your toes over head and shoulders. (This places too much weight on the bones of the neck and can injure the spine.)

    (d) Toe touches, or bending forward from the waist in a standing position. (This is not a normal stretching exercise; it places great stress on the connective tissues of the spine and can result in a painful back injury.)

3. Do not stretch injured muscles or joints. Particularly if you have injuries, see your doctor before starting an exercise program.

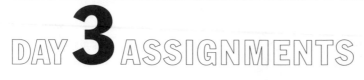 DAY **3** ASSIGNMENTS

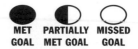

PHYSICAL VITALITY

○ 1. Improve your time for the measured mile by 2 seconds. **Time:**_____
○ 2. Do all the flexibility and stretching exercises.

NUTRITIONAL VITALITY

○ 3. Decrease total fat intake to 10% of total calories.
○ 4. Eat at least 7 half-cup portions of fruits and vegetables.

MENTAL VITALITY

○ 5. Spend at least 10 minutes practicing any deep relaxation technique.
○ 6. Complete the questionnaires in this section of the book.

EMOTIONAL & SPIRITUAL VITALITY

MEDICAL VITALITY

MANAGING STRESS   DAY 3

Everyone has a spot in the body, a special "target organ," that cries out when stress is too great. The stomach reacts with acid, the heart with angina or the breathing passages with asthma. The symptoms may be different for each person, but the process is the same and so is the message: STOP THE STRESS.

Many people don't even realize that they are having these symptoms. The problems creep up so gradually and are so constant that they accept these changes as the "normal" way to feel. The link between symptoms and stress is completely missed.

What is stress doing to you? Check the list of symptoms below to see how many you are experiencing. If any of these symptoms are a problem for you and stress is triggering them, a solution may be near. It's important to note that each of these symptoms can be caused by a medical disorder. If you have any of the symptoms listed, don't assume they are due to stress unless your doctor has ruled out the possibility that an underlying medical disorder is causing them.

Now review the list to see if there is a pattern to your symptoms. If the words "often" and "yes" are circled many times, there's a good chance that stress is responsible—at least in part—for the way you are feeling.

COMMON STRESS SIGNALS				
Symptom	**How Often It Occurs**			**At Times of Stress?**
Anger	Never	Sometimes	Often	Yes No
Backache	Never	Sometimes	Often	Yes No
Cough	Never	Sometimes	Often	Yes No
Excessive sweating	Never	Sometimes	Often	Yes No
Fatigue	Never	Sometimes	Often	Yes No
Frequent urination	Never	Sometimes	Often	Yes No
Headache	Never	Sometimes	Often	Yes No
Hyperventilation	Never	Sometimes	Often	Yes No
Impotence	Never	Sometimes	Often	Yes No
Insomnia	Never	Sometimes	Often	Yes No
Itching	Never	Sometimes	Often	Yes No
Nail biting	Never	Sometimes	Often	Yes No
Rapid heart rate	Never	Sometimes	Often	Yes No
Stomachache	Never	Sometimes	Often	Yes No

HOW MUCH STRESS DO YOU HAVE IN YOUR LIFE?

It's almost impossible to live in today's complicated world without some sources of stress. But many people are unaware how great a load they are carrying. Take a moment now to measure your current "stress load." The results may surprise you. They may also motivate you to consider making some changes in your life.

The chart on the opposite page contains a listing of events that are commonly associated with stress. Some of the events may be happy ones, such as getting married, but they are still stressful. Adding the impact of all of these events together will give you a more accurate picture of the amount of stress in your life.

Stress Load Scale

This list includes many kinds of stressful events. The numbers in the *Value* column represent an attempt to rank the events according to their seriousness. Even if you would rank the events differently, the scale should still be helpful in assessing your overall stress load.

In the *Number* (#) column, write down how many times each event has occurred in your life during the past 12 months. Multiply that number by the number in the *Value* column to get the total *Stress Load* for each event. Add up the numbers in the *Total* column to get your *Stress Load* score for the year.

A score of:

15-19	low stress load in past year
20-29	moderate stress load in past year
30+	high stress load in past year

If your score on the *Stress Load Scale* is high (a score of 30 or above), you might be tempted to say, "So what? Why change?" Here's why:

Research studies show that your chance of suffering a serious medical problem in the next year is related to the number of stressful events you are experiencing now. Thomas Holmes, M.D., and Richard H. Rahe, M.D., at the University of Washington compiled and tested a list of stressful life events that influence health and illness. Death of a family member, a divorce, and personal injury ranked at the top of the list. As we've mentioned, positive changes proved stressful as well, including marriage and retirement. If your score is high on the *Stress Load Scale*, your risk of getting sick is greater than average, and you should be doing something to lower it. Another reason to change is that stress management offers benefits far beyond the prevention of sickness. People who know how to cope well with stress feel healthier and more in control of their lives. They feel better about themselves. And they move a giant step closer to *real* vitality.

STRESS LOAD SCALE

Life Event	#	Value			Total
Family member died	_____	x	10	=	_____
Divorced or separated	_____	x	8	=	_____
Severe injury or illness	_____	x	6	=	_____
Got married	_____	x	5	=	_____
Got fired	_____	x	5	=	_____
Retired	_____	x	5	=	_____
Serious illness in family	_____	x	5	=	_____
Pregnancy	_____	x	4	=	_____
Had sexual problems	_____	x	4	=	_____
Major business change	_____	x	4	=	_____
Major financial change	_____	x	4	=	_____
Close friend died	_____	x	4	=	_____
Changed jobs	_____	x	4	=	_____
High mortgage payments	_____	x	3	=	_____
Foreclosed upon	_____	x	3	=	_____
Child left home	_____	x	3	=	_____
Lost a good friend	_____	x	3	=	_____
Trouble with in-laws	_____	x	3	=	_____
Won important recognition	_____	x	3	=	_____
Spouse started or stopped work	_____	x	3	=	_____
Started school or graduated	_____	x	3	=	_____
Major change in residence	_____	x	3	=	_____
Stopped smoking or drinking	_____	x	2	=	_____
Started a strict diet	_____	x	2	=	_____
Trouble at work	_____	x	2	=	_____
Changed schools	_____	x	2	=	_____
Had serious trouble sleeping	_____	x	1	=	_____

PINPOINTING YOUR SOURCES OF STRESS

The things that pressure other people may be totally different from the things that bother you. So the first step in this program is to figure out what are the sources of stress for *you*. The following questionnaire can help you. For each of the potential sources of stress on the chart below, do the following:

a. Estimate how many times a week this source actually creates stress for you, and enter that number in the *Frequency* column;

b. Estimate how severe the stress is for each source based on the following scale, and enter that number in the *Degree* column:

> **Very Mild   1   2   3   4   5   Very Severe**

c. Estimate the total impact this has on your life each week by multiplying the number in the *Frequency* column by the number in the *Degree* column. Enter your answer in the *Impact* column.

Sources Of Stress	Frequency	x	Degree	=	Impact
Relationships					
Spouse					
Children					
Parents					
Other relatives					
Friends, neighbors					
Work					
Boss, co-workers					
Job satisfaction					
Environment					
Lack of recognition					
Personal					
Health problems					
Self-image					
Goals					
Sex					
Financial					

STRATEGIES FOR COPING WITH STRESS

Whatever the source of your stress, there are a number of general strategies you can apply in trying to cope with it:

1. Recognize what can be changed, accept what cannot.

2. Break big problems into little ones.

3. Eliminate as many stress sources as you can.

4. Return stress to its rightful owner.

5. Maintain a fit and healthy body.

6. Avoid predictably stressful situations.

7. Remove yourself from the source of stress.

8. Don't overreact.

9. Use relaxation techniques to cancel the ill effects of stress.

Let's discuss these strategies in more detail, along with an approach or exercise for each:

1. RECOGNIZE WHAT CAN BE CHANGED, ACCEPT WHAT CANNOT

Wishing things were different won't make them different and won't make you any more comfortable about the way things are. When nothing can alter an unpleasant or stressful situation, you will find there is a certain peace in acceptance. And much less stress.

List four stressful situations in your life that you know you cannot change. Indicate next to each whether you are prepared to accept each situation as it is. Recognize, also, that your refusal to accept these unchangeable situations means that you will continue to suffer from them.

	Acceptance	
Situation	*Yes*	*No*
a. _____	❏	❏
_____		
b. _____	❏	❏
_____		
c. _____	❏	❏
_____		
d. _____	❏	❏
_____		

2. BREAK BIG PROBLEMS INTO LITTLE ONES

If the cause of your stress seems too big to tackle, break it up into manageable parts. If your home is desperately run down, you might fix it up one room at a time. If you are far behind on your bills, you might talk to your creditors about a long-term payment plan.

Use the same approach with things that make you tense. Break up your big stress-producing problems into smaller parts that create less tension and are easier to manage.

Identify two problems that feel too big to solve. Then break them down into smaller, more manageable parts. The sooner you get to work on those parts, the quicker you'll get some relief from stress.

Big Problem: _____

Smaller Parts:

    a. _____
    b. _____
    c. _____

Big Problem: _____

Smaller Parts:

    a. _____
    b. _____
    c. _____

3. ELIMINATE AS MANY STRESS SOURCES AS YOU CAN

You cannot remove all of the sources of stress in your life, but you should be able to get rid of some. Turn off the radio and stop the noise. Clear up the clutter in your life by throwing things out. And give up those stressful tasks that you volunteered for when you had extra time.

Name five stresses that you could eliminate from your life. Then do something about them. An hour spent removing these causes of stress can give you a thousand less stressful hours in the future.

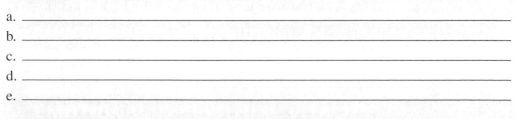

    a. _____
    b. _____
    c. _____
    d. _____
    e. _____

4. RETURN STRESS TO ITS RIGHTFUL OWNER

Have you ever noticed that some of your stress is really someone else's problem? Like the husband who repeatedly invites business associates home for dinner and expects his wife to prepare on short notice. Or the wife who serves on the boards of three community organizations and expects her husband to be at every fund-raising event. Or demanding relatives and friends who consistently burden you with their problems and expect you to come up with solutions.

The list goes on and on—if you let it. The problem stops the moment you draw the line. So draw the line! Start setting limits on the amount of stress you let other people lay on you. Here are a few suggestions that will help you return some of your stress to its rightful owner:

BE DIRECT: Don't beat around the bush. When someone is trying to lay his difficulties on you, all you have to say is, "I'm sorry things are not going well for you, and I wish I could help you, but I am burdened with my own problems and stress right now." You don't have to be mean or rude, but you must be direct. Otherwise you'll find yourself apologizing for not making their stress yours.

BE DEFINITE: If you don't want to do something, say so clearly: "No, I will not get involved. Not under any condition." A statement like that leaves little room for negotiations. You don't want to leave any room.

BE HONEST: Returning stress to its rightful owner does not mean ducking your own work or avoiding unpleasant tasks. Try to distinguish those problems that are really yours and ask the other person, "Why are you asking me to do this?" The answer to that question will make the issues very clear to you.

List three stressful burdens that other people have put on you. Write down how you will return each burden and when.

a. _____

_____

_____

_____

b. _____

_____

_____

_____

c. _____

_____

_____

_____

5. MAINTAIN A FIT AND HEALTHY BODY

The better shape you are in, the better your body will be able to tolerate the stress in your life. Your diet should be nutritious and varied, with a strong emphasis on fresh fruits and vegetables, grains, dairy products, and legumes. If you are overweight, try to change your eating habits and lifestyle to begin to slowly take off the extra weight.

Physical exercise is also important. Exercising helps release tensions of the day, and a fit body is better able to fight off stress. As you'll read in the book, exercise does not have to be strenuous to be helpful. Walking is one of the best exercises you can do.

Swimming, aerobic classes, jogging, fitness machines—all are excellent ways to keep your body in shape. The important thing is that you enjoy the activity and that you do it regularly. If you have any questions about your ability to tolerate increased physical activity, your family doctor can help you answer them.

6. AVOID PREDICTABLY STRESSFUL SITUATIONS

How many times have you put yourself voluntarily into situations that you knew for sure would upset you? Long lines in supermarkets. Busy traffic. Parties with people you don't like. It's time to recognize that most of these situations can be avoided by planning ahead (for example, shopping during off hours) and by learning how to say "no" to things you really don't want to do.

Identify the activities that trigger stress for you. Then write down how you'll avoid them in the future.

a. _____

b. _____

c. _____

d _____

e. _____

f. _____

g. _____

h. _____

7. REMOVE YOURSELF FROM THE SOURCE OF STRESS

It's impossible to remove all stress from your environment. That's why, sometimes, you've got to remove yourself. That may be very difficult when it's your job or your spouse causing the problem. But it's not impossible, and you don't have to quit your job or get a divorce to do it. You just have to learn how to slip away for a while. Take a walk into solitude. Into fresh air. Into freedom from stress.

Identify six stressful places or situations that you could get away from physically in the future and where you will go as an alternative.

Stressful place	*Alternative*
a. _____	_____
b. _____	_____
c. _____	_____
d. _____	_____
e. _____	_____
f. _____	_____

8. DON'T OVERREACT

If someone at work irritates you, a quiet conversation with that person is less stressful than quitting your job. If someone backs into your car, getting it fixed is less stressful than getting into a fight. When you react to stress with drastic measures, your reaction may often cause you more stress than the original problem.

Identify three situations that are likely to upset you in the next month. In the space below, write your normal reaction to these situations and how you will react differently the next time they arise.

Situation	*Usual Reaction*	*Planned Reaction*
a. _____	_____	_____
_____	_____	_____
_____	_____	_____
b. _____	_____	_____
_____	_____	_____
_____	_____	_____
c. _____	_____	_____
_____	_____	_____
_____	_____	_____

9. USE RELAXATION TECHNIQUES TO CANCEL THE ILL EFFECTS OF STRESS

When you cannot eliminate all sources of stress from your life, you must deal with the ill effects that stress causes. You don't have to tolerate these ill effects. You can combat them—even prevent them—through the regular use of deep relaxation techniques.

These techniques work through your nervous system to change the way your body reacts under stress. They calm your mind, release tension from your muscles, slow your heartbeat and quiet your stomach. You can use these techniques at the time stress is occurring—to help your body cancel the ill effects—or you can use them ahead of time in a preventive manner.

When you use relaxation techniques to combat the symptoms of stress, you need to begin as early as possible—as soon as the symptoms appear. If you let stress symptoms linger, the techniques will be less effective. With practice, you'll be able to recognize the earliest signs of stress and—within seconds—eliminate the discomfort by using one of these techniques.

If you use relaxation techniques often enough—even when you are not feeling stressed—you will find they induce a general calmness that acts in a preventive manner. With less than 20 minutes a day practicing these relaxation techniques, you can condition your body to defend itself against stress, and enhance your *real* vitality.

Here are four relaxation techniques. Practice each of them several times until you decide which ones are most effective for you. Then use those particular techniques regularly to protect yourself against the symptoms of stress.

Relaxation Breathing

When you are at peace with yourself, your breathing is naturally slow, deep and regular. When you are upset or stressed, your breathing rate speeds up and each breath becomes more shallow.

By controlling your breathing deliberately at times of stress, you can return your breathing to normal and induce a state of calm. You can actually use your breathing to quiet your mind, ease your stress and relax your body.

To perform this technique: Lie down in a comfortable position. Take a long, slow inhalation through your nose, filling your abdomen and lungs. Then, purse your lips and let the air slowly escape. Repeat the process, slowing your breathing with each breath until you find a pace that is most relaxing for you.

Progressive Muscle Relaxation

Your muscles are a perfect target organ for stress—they react to stress by tensing up. They convert the tension in your life to tension in your body. The car breaks down and you clench your jaw. The roof leaks and you make a fist. The kids are noisy and you arch your back. All over your body, your muscles react to stress by getting tense. The more stress in your life, the more tense your muscles become. But if you get rid of the tension in your muscles, some of the tension in your life will disappear, too. The progressive muscle relaxation technique will give you a method for releasing that tension. It is based on the principle that the best way to make a muscle relax is to contract it first. This technique works because nature's automatic response to contraction is total relaxation.

To begin, lie on your back or sit in a comfortable chair. Then close your eyes and squeeze the muscles of your face and brow as tightly as you can. Hold this position for a moment, and then relax. Repeat this process with the muscles of your jaw, neck, shoulders, abdomen, buttocks, fists, arms, legs and feet.

Guided Imagery

Guided imagery is a technique that uses mental pictures to produce deep relaxation. If you use it regularly, you can condition yourself to the point where the mere thought of a particular scene can quickly cancel some of the unpleasant effects of stress.

Lie down or sit comfortably. Close your eyes and take a few relaxation breaths. As you breathe in, say to yourself silently, "I am." As you breathe out, say, "Relaxed." Repeat, "I am...relaxed...." With your mind's eye, take a journey to the sea, to a mountaintop, or to your favorite nature spot. Feel the warmth of the sun, smell the fresh air, and feel the gentle breeze. Be in this place, feeling all the sensations of the environment and listening to the sounds. The more you concentrate on these sensations, the more you are in this place. Tell yourself this place is real. Let yourself feel how relaxed you are. When you have gone through this exercise fully, and feel relaxed and refreshed, slowly let yourself return to the present time and place.

After you have practiced the guided imagery technique, try some relaxation-inducing images of your own. Pick a scene that is especially relaxing to you and visit it mentally as often as you can.

Meditation: The Relaxation Response

Meditation is the ultimate exercise in concentration. It produces a number of changes in your body, along with a deep state of relaxation. Many people report that the calming effects of meditation last far beyond the sessions themselves.

Lie down or sit comfortably. Close your eyes and take several relaxation breaths. Focus on something in your mind—a white dot, a word, or an image. As your thoughts wander, keep returning to your focus. Do this exercise for five to twenty minutes.

It may be helpful to find a sound that you can use during your meditation training. This sound (or tone) will give you a point on which to focus your concentration. After you have practiced this routine, you may want to use other sounds or repeat a sound or word silently to yourself. (A silently repeated sound or word is known as a *mantra*.)

To achieve the complete relaxation response, you must practice meditation over and over again. Ideally, meditation routines should be performed twice a day, for at least ten minutes each time.

KEEPING A STRESS DIARY

A diary is a valuable tool when you are trying to identify where your stress is coming from and what you need to do to overcome it. The diary forces you to think more about what is happening to you and helps you recognize stressful events that might otherwise escape your attention.

For the next two weeks, use the *Stress Diary* to accurately monitor your stress level and correlate it with the events in your life. This will reveal if your stress occurs in a predictable pattern—for example, at a particular time of day, at a particular location, or when you're around a particular person.

There are three ways to use the diary:

1. At bedtime, take a moment to review the events of your day and complete the diary page.
2. Make an entry every hour or two while you are awake. This takes a lot more effort, but it will give you the most accurate picture of how much stress you are experiencing each day.
3. Make an entry every time you feel stressed. Use this time also to take a few relaxation breaths or to use a relaxation technique to control the effects of stress.

You can also use your diary to record your relaxation training sessions. Circle the time period during which you use the relaxation techniques. You should begin to see a lowering of your stress level in the time periods that follow. If you begin to use relaxation techniques regularly, you may see your stress level stay down, even if the amount of stress in your life remains high.

A FINAL NOTE

We all have different sources of stress and different ways of reacting to them. So—ultimately—you need a program that is uniquely tailored to fit your specific needs. You can create that program by adapting the basic *Stress Management Program* you have just completed. Keep using those techniques that worked well for you, and eliminate the ones that are inappropriate.

Make stress management an important priority for the rest of your life. Stop stress before it happens. Deal with it more effectively when it does occur. Cancel the ill effects when you cannot avoid the stress. And enjoy how it contributes to your *real* vitality.

Copy this diary page to create your own two-week *Stress Diary*.

STRESS DIARY

Day _____

Hour	Stress Level	Cause Of Stress
12–2 am	0 1 2 3 4 5	
2–4	0 1 2 3 4 5	
4–6	0 1 2 3 4 5	
6–8	0 1 2 3 4 5	
8–10	0 1 2 3 4 5	
10–12	0 1 2 3 4 5	
12–2 pm	0 1 2 3 4 5	
2–4	0 1 2 3 4 5	
4–6	0 1 2 3 4 5	
6–8	0 1 2 3 4 5	
8–10	0 1 2 3 4 5	
10–12	0 1 2 3 4 5	

Stress Level: 0 = No stress; completely calm
1 = Minimal stress; relaxed
2 = Slight stress; slightly anxious
3 = Moderate stress; anxious
4 = High stress; very anxious
5 = Severe stress; extremely anxious

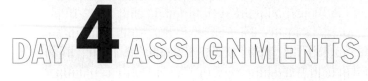

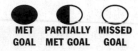

MET · PARTIALLY · MISSED
GOAL · MET GOAL · GOAL

PHYSICAL VITALITY

1. Improve your time for the measured mile by 2 seconds.   **Time:**_____
2. Do all the flexibility and stretching exercises.

NUTRITIONAL VITALITY

3. Decrease total fat intake to 10% of total calories.
4. Eat at least 7 half-cup portions of fruits and vegetables.

MENTAL VITALITY

5. Spend at least 10 minutes practicing any deep relaxation technique.
6. Identify and eliminate as many sources of stress in your life as you can.

EMOTIONAL & SPIRITUAL VITALITY

MEDICAL VITALITY

AEROBIC EXERCISE

DAY 4

Many people think that the primary benefit of aerobic fitness is the ability to participate in high-intensity exercise, such as jogging or aerobic dancing. But the advantages of being aerobically fit go far beyond that definition. Aerobic fitness allows you to take part in most activities without excessive strain on your cardiovascular system and without "losing your breath." It will also improve the quality of your life, and it may increase the length of your life. Specifically, its benefits include:

- **Reduced risk of heart attack and stroke:** People who are aerobically fit have a reduced risk of heart attack and stroke. Their risk is reduced, in part, because their heart muscle becomes more efficient at contracting and pumping blood, so more blood (and oxygen) is delivered with each beat and their resting heart rate is lower. Aerobic fitness also has an effect on the skeletal muscles that are used during exercise, so they become more efficient in their use of energy and require less oxygen to perform the same amount of work. Aerobic exercise increases the blood level of HDL cholesterol—the so-called "good cholesterol"—which, in turn, reduces the risk of coronary heart disease. Regular aerobic exercise also lowers the blood pressure and protects against the development of hypertension, which is yet another risk factor for coronary heart disease and stroke.

- **Reduced risk of obesity and diabetes:** People who do aerobic exercise regularly burn more calories than sedentary individuals and thus have a lower risk of obesity. A person who burns calories this way on a regular basis significantly reduces his or her risk of developing Type II diabetes (commonly referred to as "adult-onset"). During an aerobic workout, your body burns calories faster as your muscles work harder. Not only are more calories burned during the activity itself, but aerobic exercise also causes your metabolism to maintain a more rapid rate for some time afterward. Studies have shown that a person's metabolic rate can remain elevated for 20 minutes to an hour after exercise. Aerobics also activate enzyme systems in the muscles that prevent insulin resistance, which further protects against the development of diabetes.

- **Reduced risk of cancer:** In a study reported in 1994 in the *Journal of the National Cancer Institute*, researchers analyzed more than 1,000 women ages 40 and younger, half of whom had early breast cancer. The study found that women who exercised one to three hours a week had about a 30 percent reduced risk of developing breast cancer, compared to women who were not active. Women who exercised for four hours a week or more were at least 50 percent less likely to develop the disease. Some investigators believe that this positive effect of physical activity may be related to its ability to interfere with ovulation and thus cut down a woman's exposure to the female hormones (estrogen, progesterone) that stimulate the growth of breast cells. Regular physical activity also reduces the risk of colon cancer, probably by speeding the transit time of potential carcinogens through the intestinal tract.

- **Increased endurance:** Aerobically fit individuals are able to complete their normal activities more easily and with less fatigue. They are able to perform strenuous activities for long periods of time without feeling exhausted. Aerobic training increases the amount of physical work they can do, and speeds their recovery afterward. Aerobic exercise also increases the efficiency of the heart, so it does not have to beat as rapidly to get the same task done.

- **Enhanced sense of well-being:** People who do aerobic exercise regularly say it gives them a sense of accomplishment as their fitness level improves, and makes them feel more competent and confident about themselves generally. Aerobic exercise also causes the brain to release chemicals called endorphins, which produce an enhanced sense of well-being in most individuals. In some people, the endorphins actually create a state of euphoria. Physical activity also provides an extremely effective way to release tension and control the effects of stress. Your exercise activities will take you away from some of the boring routines of daily living and generate new opportunities for pleasant social contact.

- **Decreased overall mortality risk:** Years ago, a landmark study of about 17,000 Harvard graduates indicated that men who burned 2,000 calories a week in physical activities—the equivalent of approximately one hour of brisk walking every day— slashed their death rates from all causes by a remarkable 28 percent, compared to a group of their Harvard peers who didn't exercise.

HOW TO DEVELOP AEROBIC FITNESS

Any activity that forces you to breathe deeply and use your major muscles in a continuous and rhythmic fashion can be used to improve aerobic fitness. To achieve cardiovascular fitness, you need to work out for at least 20 minutes, four times a week, at an intensity level high enough to raise your heart rate to 60 to 90 percent of its maximum. (Your maximum heart rate is determined by subtracting your age from 220. For example: If you are 40 years old, your maximum heart rate is 180; so you should exercise in the range of 108 to 162 beats per minute to remain in your target zone of 60 to 90 percent of maximum.) Recent research, however, indicates that while you need to exercise continuously for 20 or more minutes to fully achieve aerobic fitness, your body can still benefit from briefer periods of activity, and at the same time, you'll gradually be able to build up to a more vigorous exercise program. Particularly if you haven't exercised for weeks, months or longer, and need to get back in shape, moderate activities like short walks through the neighborhood, using the stairs instead of the elevator to go up a flight or two, or even an hour of gardening can help improve your fitness level. (Some people call activities like these "Exercise Lite.")

Keep in mind that eventually your goal should be to incorporate a more intensive exercise program into your life, and enjoy the full cardiovascular benefits of an aerobic workout. But to begin, just get moving. You'll start to experience how enjoyable physical activity can be, and how much better it can make you feel. In this program, walking and/or running are the primary activities you'll monitor, but there are many other aerobic activities you can use to build and maintain your fitness level. In the material that follows, you will find information about several excellent aerobic activities. Try as many of them as you can before settling into a program that includes all of your favorites on a regular basis. It's a very good idea to mix activities—not only to prevent boredom, but also because you'll be using different muscles in each activity, which will improve your overall fitness level.

HOW TO ACCOMPLISH YOUR AEROBIC ASSIGNMENTS

In this program, walking and/or running are our primary aerobic activities. Each day, you will be asked to walk or run one mile after a brief series of stretching exercises.

Your first task is to find a measured track or measure out a mile on your own. Most high school and recreation facilities have a quarter-mile track. If you measure the mile yourself—by using your car's odometer, for example— do it on a flat road with as few interruptions (e.g., stop lights) as possible.

Beginning with your assignment on Day 1, walk or run the mile at a brisk (but not exhausting) pace, and time yourself with a watch to the nearest second. You should be able to pass the "talk test" as you walk, meaning you should be a little short of breath but should still be able to carry on a conversation.

On each of the subsequent days of the program, you should cover the mile at a slightly faster pace than you did the day before. For example, with an eye on your watch, aim toward walking (or running) two to three seconds faster tomorrow than you do today; then cut another two to three seconds the following day, and so on. By the end of the four weeks, you will have reduced your overall walking (or running) time by one minute, while still covering the same one-mile distance.

Of course, each day you may not precisely hit the two-to-three-second target. But with your watch as your guide, make small adjustments in your pace and stride, and you'll come very close. Also, use landmarks along your walking or running route to help monitor your speed. Gradually increase the energy you put into each stride, and swing your arms actively. Keep your head up, your eyes off the ground, and back erect.

Walking

Walking is an ideal aerobic activity. It's easy to do, doesn't require expensive equipment or facilities, isn't limited by your age or geographic location, and doesn't require professional instruction or supervision. Walking will improve your aerobic fitness level if you maintain a pace brisk enough to get your heart rate in the target zone—60 to 90 percent of the maximum.

Walking was neglected as a fitness activity until recently because many people incorrectly believed that it wasn't strenuous enough to raise the heart rate to the levels needed to produce cardiovascular conditioning. Besides, many people found it hard to believe that an exercise as simple, easy and comfortable as walking could be that good for your health. The research now shows that almost all people can get their heart rates up into the "conditioning zone" by walking. And the "no pain, no gain" way of thinking has given way to common sense.

Regular walking enhances your endurance by increasing the capacity of your lungs to move air in and out and by improving the strength and efficiency of the muscles in your legs, abdomen, and back. An additional benefit of walking is that people who are out of shape or overweight can walk a mile more easily than they can run it. For aerobic fitness, walking fits the bill perfectly.

Walking can be done at a number of levels, ranging from an easy stroll (about one to two miles per hour) to striding or race walking (about five miles per hour). A good pace to shoot for is three to four miles per hour.

One of the goals of our program is to help you to comfortably and safely increase your walking speed. This goal goes hand-in-hand with increasing your aerobic fitness level.

In today's assignment, we'll show you how to do it.

CHOOSING WALKING SHOES

More than anything else you can buy, a good pair of walking shoes will add comfort and safety to your walks. The uppers should be made of material that breathes (leather or nylon mesh) so your feet don't overheat. The heel and sole should have extra cushioning to absorb the shock of hitting the ground. The sole should be designed with a "rocker profile." (This makes a heel-to-toe motion happen even more easily than normal.) The heel counter (the back of the shoe that cups your heel) should be firm enough to hold the back of your foot well, and the heel collar (the top of the counter) should be well-padded for comfort. Your arch should be well-supported (you'll be able to feel it), and there should be enough room in the front of the shoe for you to wiggle your toes a little.

Even with good walking shoes, you'll want to treat your feet with special care. Wear light socks that fit just right—neither too tight nor too loose. Use cotton or cotton/orlon blends, which help to carry moisture away from your skin.

Running

Obviously, running places more demands on your body than walking, making the aerobic workout more intense. If your beginning fitness level is low—you've been inactive for years—you'll be better off starting with a walking program. But for people who are already at an appropriate fitness level, running is an excellent choice. However, keep in mind that your goal is to cover a distance of one mile, whether you're walking or running. A significant drawback to running is the increased risk of injury, especially to the knees and joints. Joggers need to take particular care in selecting shoes that provide support while absorbing shock.

Swimming And Other Water Exercises

Swimming is one of the best exercises for overall body conditioning. It is also one of the safer aerobic exercise choices. Swimming is an impact-free activity; it does not stress bones and joints. Also, unlike running, walking, and cycling, swimming builds upper body strength. What's more, many people associate water and swimming pools with fun, so they are more likely to stick with a swimming program.

Besides swimming, other aerobic exercises that can be done in water include water walking and water aerobics. Water walking—which involves walking from one side of a pool's shallow end to the other against the resistance that the water provides—is an excellent way to condition leg muscles. In water aerobics, people do repetitive leg and arm movements while standing in the water. Check with your local YMCA or public pool to see if they offer these classes.

Cycling

Riding a bicycle is another effective aerobic exercise. It raises your heart rate and develops lower body strength. Cycling also offers the pleasures of changing scenery, fresh air, and a sense of speed. But the risk of injury is much higher than with some other aerobic activities, especially if you ride through busy city streets. In some locations (like city streets) bicyclists must stop frequently, so the aerobic benefits are impeded. If you choose bicycling as your aerobic activity, be sure to wear a good helmet and plan a route through safe, less traveled roads.

Aerobics Classes

Most health clubs offer a variety of aerobics classes, including aerobic dance, low-impact aerobics, and step aerobics. All involve performing repetitive movements—such as arm swings, leg lifts, and dance steps—to the beat of rhythmic music. Low-impact classes reduce the risk of leg strain and injury because in all the moves, at least one foot remains on the floor. Step aerobics, which are mostly low-impact movement, use low benches, roughly 4 to 12 inches high, to accentuate the aerobic and muscle-building effect of the movements.

Many people are stimulated by the energetic atmosphere and group support of aerobics classes. You may find the sheer fun of dancing to music so exhilarating that the exercise becomes not only physically beneficial but also emotionally uplifting and satisfying. If you decide to start taking aerobics classes, make sure you find a reputable health club or dance studio staffed by certified instructors.

Stationary Exercise Machines

Stationary machines—bicycles, rowing machines, stair climbers, treadmills, cross-country ski simulators—are another fine choice for aerobic exercise. They provide most of the benefits of the original activity they are modeled after, but offer an added advantage: You don't have to contend with real-world obstacles, such as foul weather, traffic, and stoplights. Also, if you have a machine at home, you can work out while watching television or listening to music.

Exercise Videotapes

Since the video exercise boom started in the 1980s, literally hundreds of home exercise programs have been produced. It seems as though every major—and minor—star in Hollywood has come out with a tape in the last few years. Most of these programs are designed and overseen by professionals in the exercise field, so the risk of injury is minimal.

Most video stores rent exercise tapes, so you can try them before committing to a purchase. It's a good idea to purchase several different exercise videos so you can vary your routines. Be sure to purchase programs that are appropriate to your current fitness level. Don't worry about outgrowing them as your fitness level improves. You can always use your easier programs on days when you want a lighter workout.

The table on page 64 will help you compare the amount of calories you can burn with various aerobic activities.

The Warm-Up and Cool-Down

Among the most important parts of any aerobic program is the warm-up, a period of mild activity before you begin walking that will help your heart get gradually "up to speed." It also prepares your muscles and joints for the activity that follows, which helps prevent injuries during the most vigorous part of your activity.

Some people skip the warm-up before a fitness walk because they think that walking is not intense enough an exercise to warrant the time. Skipping the warm-up is a mistake because you interfere with the benefits of the walk and expose yourself to unnecessary risk of injury. Besides, the warm-up is more than a physical activity—it's a time to get your mind relaxed and in tune with the coming walk.

There are two parts to the warm-up: A 3- to 5-minute period of walking or marching in place that starts slowly and gradually increases in intensity, and then some stretching that will prepare your muscles for your exercise session, concentrating on those muscles that will be worked most heavily as you walk or run. The stretching exercises on pages 37-38 were specifically chosen because of their suitability for use before and after walking or jogging.

A proper cool-down is essential after a vigorous aerobic workout. It helps you avoid the problems that can occur when you suddenly go from being very active to standing still, and it can improve the way you feel for the rest of the day. There are two elements to the ideal cool-down: A period of gradually decreasing movement and a stretching session.

Gradually decreasing your movement allows your heart to return more slowly to its normal resting rate, and prevents feelings of faintness that can occur if blood "pools" in your legs. The simplest way to prevent blood "pooling" in your legs is to decrease your speed gradually over a 3- to 5-minute period, until your pace is down to a stroll.

Stretching again the muscles that have been worked and stressed the most during your walk will keep them from being sore afterward. The best time to stretch is immediately after the cool-down. The stretching exercises in Day 2 can be used in both the warm-up and cool-down.

AEROBICS FOR YOUR HEART

After four weeks of aerobic exercise—regular walking, for example—you'll probably find that even though you're walking faster, the walking itself is getting easier. That's because your body is becoming aerobically conditioned. Your heart muscle is getting stronger and pumping blood more efficiently. As a result, more blood is delivered with each heartbeat, so your heart can beat more slowly and still supply enough blood to your body. Because of this conditioning process, your heart rate will not speed up as much as it did when you first started exercising, and your breathing will be easier and more regular.

As your physical condition continues to improve, walking will undoubtedly become more comfortable and more pleasant. A feeling of comfort with the walking pace you have set for yourself is a signal to continue to cut two to three seconds a day from your time by increasing your walking speed. Although walking slowly burns up as many calories as walking quickly over the same distance, increasing your pace offers you an additional benefit: It further improves your level of aerobic fitness.

Remember, to build aerobic conditioning you should strive to keep your heart rate between 60 and 90 percent of its maximum (see page 56 for how to estimate your maximum heart rate). Increasing your speed is the simplest way to bring your heart rate back up if conditioning has allowed it to drop below the target zone. But increases should be made gradually (by two to three seconds a day) and carefully, to avoid overexerting yourself and raising your heart rate too high. Here's a safe way to do it: At regular intervals (perhaps weekly), check to see if your heart rate has fallen below your target zone. Five or ten minutes into your walk, stop and measure your pulse. Place your index and middle fingers over the artery in your wrist (see diagram). Count the number of beats, or "pulses," you feel in 30 seconds. Multiply this number by two to determine the number of times your heart is beating each minute.

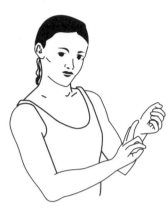

If your heart rate is below 60 percent of its maximum, you can increase your walking speed ever more slightly and measure your pulse again after five minutes. If the faster pace raises your heart rate back up in the target zone, complete your walk at this new speed. If your heart rate is still too low, increase your speed a little more and recheck your pulse a few minutes later.

If your heart rate *exceeds* the 90 percent target level, then you need to slow down, even if it means not adhering to the two or three second-per-day reduction in your time for the mile. Once your body becomes better conditioned, your heart rate should fall into the target zone, and you can begin cutting time off your mile again.

MAKING YOUR COMMITMENT TO EXERCISE

People often complain that they don't have enough time for exercise in their busy schedules. The real truth is that they haven't made aerobic exercise a priority. We all can find time for things that are important to us. And when you are prepared to say that exercise is an important priority, you *will* find time to do it.

Here's a list of some of the most popular excuses for not exercising, along with some ways to overcome them:

I didn't get enough sleep, and I'm too tired to exercise. Exercise is the best thing you can do for your energy level when you're tired. Aerobic exercise will revitalize you, whereas sitting around will only compound your fatigue.

Some people try to avoid exercising when they haven't gotten enough sleep, because they find exercise more difficult to do when they're tired. The fact is, after a poor night's sleep, your legs may feel heavier and more sluggish than usual. But tiredness is not a good reason to skip your aerobic workout. Just expect a little less from yourself and adjust your workout accordingly. If you usually walk briskly, go a little slower. Setting limited goals on these days will make it easier to get started, and a partial workout is always preferable to no workout at all.

I'm expecting a phone call, so I can't leave the house. There's almost always a reason you need to be home—whether it's a phone call you're expecting, a delivery you're waiting for, or a repair person who's working in the house. Schedule your calls before or after your workout. Make appointments for home repairs at times that won't interfere with your exercise plans. If you're expecting a package, leave a note authorizing the delivery person to leave the parcel at the door so you don't have to wait at home for it.

It upsets my stomach to exercise after I eat. If exercising after eating makes you uncomfortable, set up your schedule so your aerobic workouts always precede your meals (consider making exercise the very first thing you do after you wake up). If you happen to be hungry when it's time to exercise, try a light snack like half an apple or a piece of toast to tide you over until after your workout.

I've got appointments from early in the morning until late at night. Many people are so busy with work, they have little time to do anything else—let alone exercise. You'll always find time to exercise, however—if it's important enough to you.

The best way to get around this problem is to schedule walking as your first appointment every day. Start scheduling the rest of your day only after you've set aside time to exercise. Don't make the mistake of trying to squeeze your walking into the empty blocks of time that remain in your schedule. Those empty blocks have a way of disappearing, leaving you disappointed and out of shape.

I had to travel to another city, and it's not safe to walk where the hotel is located. Travel can present many excuses for not exercising—from the safety of the neighborhood surrounding your hotel to the fact that you "forgot" your workout clothes at home. But travel excuses can all be avoided with a little planning. One of the most helpful strategies is to stay at a hotel that offers access to workout facilities. Most larger hotels now have fitness facilities on-site; others have agreements with nearby gyms. Such arrangements solve your safety concerns and eliminate the "weather" excuse as you're guaranteed good weather indoors.

It's raining, so I can't walk. Ordinarily, we go to great effort to keep ourselves dry, usually for good reasons (we're dressed for work, for example). But there's no need to stay dry when you exercise (you head straight for the shower, anyway, after you exercise). So, if it's just drizzling (and a big storm isn't looming), you should consider exercising outdoors anyway. You'll stay warm and relatively dry if you wear a vinyl or gortex outer layer and one or more soft inner layers. Wear a baseball cap or visor to keep the rain out of your eyes.

If it's raining heavily, it's probably a good idea to stay indoors. (If you get very wet while exercising in cold weather, your body temperature can drop dangerously low.) Prepare ahead for rainy days with indoor exercise alternatives. Among the aerobic choices you should consider are: Using a video exercise program; walking in an enclosed shopping mall; purchasing a one-day lesson at a local fitness facility; going out for an evening of dancing—or staying in and dancing to your favorite music. By the way, all of these are good choices when it's extremely hot outside, too.

APPROXIMATE CALORIES BURNED DURING VARIOUS ACTIVITIES

(calories burned per minute)

Activity	Weight			
	130 lb	**150 lb**	**170 lb**	**200 lb**
Basketball	8.0	9.5	11.0	12.5
Carpentry	3.0	3.5	4.0	5.0
Car wash and wax	3.5	4.0	4.5	5.0
Cleaning	4.0	4.5	5.0	6.0
Football	8.0	9.0	10.0	12.0
Gardening	3.0-8.0	4.0-9.0	4.0-10.0	5.0-12.0
Golf	5.0	6.0	7.0	8.0
Hiking	7.0	8.5	9.5	10.5
Horseback riding (trot)	6.5	7.5	8.5	10.0
Jumping rope (80 jumps/min)	10.0	11.0	12.5	14.5
Mowing lawn (hand mower)	6.5	7.5	8.5	9.5
Racquetball	10.5	12.0	13.5	16.5
Running (6 mph)	7.0	8.0	9.0	10.0
Shoveling snow	7.0	8.0	9.0	11.0
Skating	7.0	8.0	9.0	11.0
Skiing	7.0	8.0	9.0	11.0
Squash	12.5	14.0	16.0	19.5
Stair climbing	6.0	7.0	8.0	10.0
Tennis	6.5	7.5	8.5	10.0
Walking (3 mph)	3.5	4.0	4.5	5.0
Walking (4 mph)	5.0	6.0	6.5	7.5

It's too cold out. You're unlikely to get too cold exercising outdoors if you dress properly. The key steps to take: Protect your hands with gloves or mittens; wear a hat to prevent loss of body heat from your head; and layer your clothes. (You can remove an outer layer if you get too hot.)

Cold weather can present some interesting aerobic exercise opportunities—cross-country skiing and snowshoeing, for example. Just walking through the snow can be fun (and excellent exercise) provided you have the proper footwear. If you live in a particularly cold environment, consider purchasing a seasonal gym membership. A gym will provide you with a warm workout haven on the coldest days of winter (or those days you just can't face the outdoors) and you can fulfill your aerobic assignment by walking on a treadmill.

It's too hot out. Hot weather can be just as bad for your exercise routine as cold weather, if not worse. The thought of expending more energy than you absolutely have to on a hot day is never an appealing one. But there are a number of things you can do to maintain (and enjoy) your exercise routine through the summer.

Schedule your aerobic workouts very early in the morning or in the evening (before it gets dark) to avoid the hottest times of the day. Wear clothing that is lightweight and loose-fitting. Your best fabric choices are those that breathe, including cotton, nylon, and polypropylene. Avoid all rubberized clothing; it traps moisture and heat, and can cause your body temperature to rise dangerously. Use hot weather as an excuse to try out new types of exercise like swimming and water aerobics. Also, look for indoor exercise opportunities in buildings that are air-conditioned.

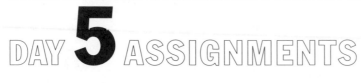

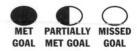

MET   PARTIALLY   MISSED
GOAL   MET GOAL   GOAL

PHYSICAL VITALITY

1. Improve your time for the measured mile by 2 seconds.   **Time:**_____
2. Do all the flexibility and stretching exercises.
3. Do chest, back and arm strength training exercises.

NUTRITIONAL VITALITY

4. Decrease total fat intake to 10% of total calories.
5. Eat at least 7 half-cup portions of fruits and vegetables.

MENTAL VITALITY

6. Spend at least 10 minutes practicing any deep relaxation technique.
7. Identify and eliminate as many sources of stress in your life as you can.

EMOTIONAL & SPIRITUAL VITALITY

MEDICAL VITALITY

STRENGTH TRAINING
DAY 5

Strength training occurs when your muscles work against resistance to increase their tone and strength. It is an important component of your program for total vitality.

Strength training can be done by virtually anyone, no matter what his or her age, and at little or no cost. Along the way, it has both physical and mental benefits. On the physical side, this form of exercise can increase your muscle mass and the strength of your connective tissue, improve balance and coordination, and enhance your bone strength. Also, as strength training builds stronger muscles, it leaves these muscles less vulnerable to injuries. Even if injuries occur, you are more likely to recover from them quickly.

By increasing your lean muscle mass, strength training can also "rev up" your metabolism. As that happens, you'll burn more calories—not simply while you're exercising, but throughout the day, even while you're sitting or sleeping.

On the psychological side, strength training can increase your feelings of self-confidence as it helps you accomplish some of your vitality goals. As you notice your body getting stronger, you'll feel more motivated to adhere to the program.

Here are brief descriptions of some recent studies that have clearly demonstrated the benefits of strength training:

- In a study at Tufts University and Pennsylvania State University, a group of sedentary, postmenopausal women who were placed on a strength-training program for a year experienced increases in bone density in their spine and hips—protection against the development of osteoporosis—while a comparison group of non-trainers experienced a loss of bone density.

- Researchers at the University of Maryland and the National Institutes of Aging found that a group of men working out on a strength-training program for 16 weeks experienced not only substantial improvements in both upper and lower body strength, but also an increase in muscle mass and a decrease in body fat.

- A group of men and women (ages 65 to 79) were evaluated by University of Vermont investigators before and after 12 weeks of strength training; at the end of the study period, these volunteers not only had stronger muscles, but they had better endurance and were able to exercise aerobically for longer periods of time.

Strength training, then, can add to your *real* vitality, overall conditioning, and quality of life. It can help you maintain—even increase—muscle and bone strength, prevent injuries, and reduce your risk of backaches. And psychologically, it helps create feelings of well-being and self-confidence.

There are other advantages to strength training. Without it, your muscle strength will dip modestly beginning in your thirties, and then that loss will accelerate more significantly in your fifties and beyond. As that wasting of muscle occurs, it causes potentially serious problems in everyday living, particularly among the elderly. For example, routine tasks like carrying grocery bags and opening windows—even walking up and down a few steps—can become difficult. Also, as the joints and bones weaken, the likelihood of falls and fractures increases. Strengthening exercises, however, can halt and actually reverse that loss of muscle strength, even among men and women in their eighties and nineties.

In a single chapter, it is not possible to present an entire strength-training regimen for your entire body. This chapter will introduce you to the concept of strength training, and provide some exercises that show you what's possible with just a few minutes a week of this type of physical activity. You'll be pleasantly surprised by the amount of progress you can make in 28 days; I hope this will motivate you to integrate strength training into your life for the long-term.

These exercises do not require you to invest in weightlifting equipment or join a health club (although you might choose to do so down the road). They will work your major muscle groups simply by using your own body weight to provide the resistance needed to build strength.

Here are some guidelines to keep in mind while you integrate these strength-training exercises into your vitality program:

- To begin, use these exercises twice a week, performing the minimum number of repetitions per exercise.

- Once you're able to do the minimum number of repetitions (for example, 10 repetitions for the standard push-ups), increase the amount of resistance by doing one or more of the following:

  - Raise the number of repetitions.

  - Increase the number of sets of each exercise.

  - Reduce the rest time between each set or exercise.

  - Adapt the exercises to make them more challenging. (For example, try doing a one-footed push-up which will increase your instability and increase the difficulty of the exercise.)

STRENGTH TRAINING DO'S AND DON'TS

Do's

1. Always do a general warm-up routine first.

2. Always stretch the muscles beforehand that will be involved in your strengthening routine.

3. Use progressive resistance. The strength of a muscle will continue to improve only if the muscle is made to work progressively harder.

4. Use short sets that are repeated later. An efficient way to improve strength is to allow brief rest periods between bouts of vigorous exercise.

5. Perform all strengthening exercises in a slow and controlled manner.

6. Exhale during the exertion phase of each repetition.

7. If you do exercises to strengthen the muscles on one side of a joint (for example, the biceps), also exercise to strengthen the muscles on the opposite side (the triceps).

8. Start and finish each exercise in a "neutral spine" posture. The ears, shoulders, hips, knees and ankles should all be in a straight vertical line, from top to bottom, as though a plumb line were running from the ears to the ankles. This position keeps your body in the best possible alignment.

Don'ts

1. Do not do large numbers of repetitions with low resistance. This type of exercising will produce an uncomfortable burning sensation in the muscles, but will not produce any significant improvement in strength.

2. Do not hold your breath while exercising.

3. Do not perform strengthening exercises on the same muscles on consecutive days.

LEGS/GLUTES - Lunge

With your legs shoulder-width apart, head up, and back straight, step forward, bending the leg until the front thigh is parallel to the floor. DO NOT let the knee move forward over the toe. Return and alternate legs.

Complete 20-30 times.
Do 1-3 sets.

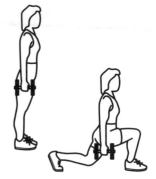

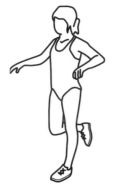

ANKLE/FOOT - One-Foot Balance

Attempt to balance on one leg. Begin with the eyes open, then try to perform the exercise with the eyes closed. Hold 20-30 seconds.

Repeat 5-8 times per set. Do 4-5 sets per session.
Do 3 sessions per week.

LEGS/QUADS - Ninety/Ninety

Position your back against a wall so that the knee joints form 90° angles. Hold for 90 seconds.

Complete 5-10 repetitions.
Do 1-3 sets.

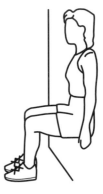

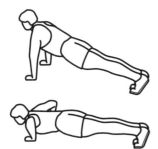

CHEST - Standard Push-Up

From a starting position with your hands less than a shoulder-width apart, and with your body straight, lower your body until your chest touches the floor.

Complete 10-20 repetitions.
Do 1-3 sets.

CHEST - Modified Push-Up

From a starting position with your knees bent, your hands more than a shoulder-width apart and with your body straight, lower your body until your chest touches the floor. Exhale as you move to the "up" position.

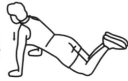

Complete 10-20 repetitions.
Do 1-3 sets.

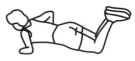

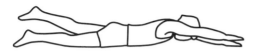

BACK - Prone Opposite Arm and Leg Lift
Keeping one knee locked, raise the leg and the opposite arm 8-10 inches from the floor. Hold for 5-15 seconds.

Repeat 5-10 times on each side.
Do 3 sessions per week.

ARMS/TRICEPS - Bench Dip
Keeping your elbows close to the sides, lower your body until your elbows are bent to a 90° angle. Exhale as you move to the "up" position.

Complete 10-15 repetitions.
Do 1-3 sets.

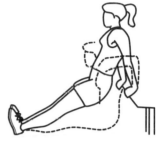

BACK - Prone on Elbows
Raise up on your elbows and raise your entire body off the floor. Only the toes and elbows should be touching. Breathe normally during this exercise. Hold 10-30 seconds.

Repeat 5-10 times.
Do 3 sessions per week.

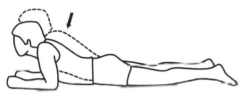
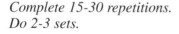

ABS - Abdominal Curl
Curl your upper body toward your knee until your shoulder blades and upper back clear the floor. Be sure to keep your chin off your chest. Exhale as you move to the "up" position.

Complete 15-30 repetitions.
Do 2-3 sets.

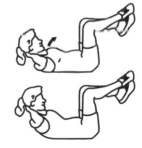

ABS - Side Crunch
With your knees bent, bend sideways at the waist, moving your shoulder towards your hip. Repeat with the other side. Do not pull on your head. Exhale as you move to the "up" position.

Complete 15-25 repetitions.
Do 1-4 sets.

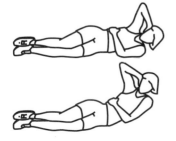

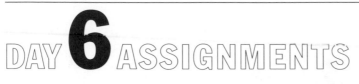

DAY **6** ASSIGNMENTS

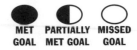

MET GOAL   PARTIALLY MET GOAL   MISSED GOAL

PHYSICAL VITALITY

1. Improve your time for the measured mile by 2 seconds.   **Time:**_____
2. Do all the flexibility and stretching exercises.
3. Do leg and abdominal strength training exercises.

NUTRITIONAL VITALITY

4. Decrease total fat intake to 10% of total calories.
5. Eat at least 7 half-cup portions of fruits and vegetables.

MENTAL VITALITY

6. Spend at least 10 minutes practicing any deep relaxation technique.
7. Identify and eliminate as many sources of stress in your life as you can.

EMOTIONAL & SPIRITUAL VITALITY

MEDICAL VITALITY

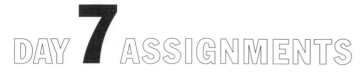

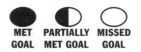

MET   PARTIALLY   MISSED
GOAL   MET GOAL   GOAL

PHYSICAL VITALITY

1. Improve your time for the measured mile by 2 seconds.   **Time:**_____

2. Do all the flexibility and stretching exercises.

NUTRITIONAL VITALITY

3. Decrease total fat intake to 10% of total calories.

4. Eat at least 7 half-cup portions of fruits and vegetables.

MENTAL VITALITY

5. Spend at least 10 minutes practicing any deep relaxation technique.

6. Identify and eliminate as many sources of stress in your life as you can.

EMOTIONAL & SPIRITUAL VITALITY

MEDICAL VITALITY

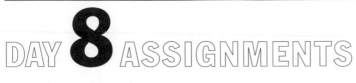

DAY 8 ASSIGNMENTS

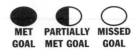

PHYSICAL VITALITY

1. Improve your time for the measured mile by 2 seconds.   **Time:**_____

2. Do all the flexibility and stretching exercises.

3. Do chest, back and arm strength training exercises.

NUTRITIONAL VITALITY

4. Decrease total fat intake to 10% of total calories.

5. Eat at least 7 half-cup portions of fruits and vegetables.

6. Supplement as necessary to reach the vitamin recommendations.

MENTAL VITALITY

7. Spend at least 10 minutes practicing any deep relaxation technique.

8. Identify and eliminate as many sources of stress in your life as you can.

EMOTIONAL & SPIRITUAL VITALITY

MEDICAL VITALITY

VITAMINS

DAY 8

Until recently, vitamins were considered important primarily for avoiding deficiency-related medical disorders. Nutrition experts recommended doses of each vitamin at a level just high enough to ward off deficiency diseases like scurvy (vitamin C), anemia (folic acid), rickets (vitamin D), and beri beri (thiamin).

But recent research has transformed the way we look at these nutrients and caused many authorities to alter their recommendations. New studies have demonstrated that certain vitamins (as well as minerals) may do much more than prevent deficiency disorders—especially when taken in large amounts. Evidence indicates that higher levels of selected nutrients may actually slow or prevent the physical deterioration associated with aging—a deterioration once considered to be inevitable. Proper supplements of vitamins and minerals may help many people prevent some of the most common chronic diseases and illnesses associated with aging—from heart disease to cancer to cataracts.

This nutritional approach is part of an entirely new way of looking at aging and health. In the past, we've assumed that our health would decline as we grew older and that the frequency, severity, and duration of our illnesses and disorders would increase. Today, many physicians believe we can significantly retard the process of aging by changing the way we eat, increasing our physical activity levels, avoiding cigarettes, limiting alcohol intake, and—yes—taking supplements of certain vitamins.

The goal of this approach is not merely to prevent disease, but to attain excellent health, or high-level wellness. The idea is that, instead of spending our early years in good health and our later years in physical decline, we'll be able to live our entire lives in good health—right up to the day we die. Will vitamin supplements alone enable us to accomplish this goal? No. But there is now good reason to believe that such supplements—in combination with a healthy lifestyle—can significantly contribute toward our achieving good health for our entire lives. The ability of vitamin supplements to help us attain excellent health makes them an important part of this overall fitness plan.

In this program, your primary vitamin goal is to make sure you're consuming at least the U.S. Recommended Daily Allowance or USRDA (also called the Reference Daily Intakes, or RDIs) for each vitamin—through food as much as possible. But later in this chapter, you will also find my own recommendations of how much of each vitamin you really need. These recommended vitamin doses are never lower than the USRDAs and are sometimes higher, because recent research suggests that higher levels of certain nutrients may help you achieve higher levels of wellness and better protect you against illness. (For a brief description of the USRDAs—and the RDAs—and who developed and issued them, see the box on page 78.)

VITAMIN BASICS

Vitamins are organic (carbon-containing) substances derived from living material (animals or plants) and are essential in small amounts for good health. They play many critical roles in the body. Among other things, they promote proper vision, blood clotting, and formation of hormones and genetic materials; maintain tissues; and strengthen the immune system. Vitamins are also important for the processing of other nutrients and for the functioning of the body's enzyme systems. We currently know about 13 vitamins.

We obtain most of these nutrients through diet, with a couple of exceptions. Your skin manufactures vitamin D when exposed to sunlight, and your body produces niacin (though somewhat inefficiently) if you consume enough of an amino acid called tryptophan.

Our knowledge about vitamins is actually relatively recent. Scientists identified the first vitamin, vitamin A, in 1913. When researchers discovered that the chemical structure of this nutrient contained an *amine* (a nitrogen-containing chemical compound), they labeled the important substance *vitamine* (an amine vital to life). The *e* was eventually dropped from the name, and these nutrients have since been referred to as vitamins.

Vitamins constitute one of several categories of nutrients necessary for normal body growth, maintenance, and tissue repair. Some nutrients—fats, carbohydrates, and proteins—are referred to as *macronutrients*; they make up most of our diet and supply the body with energy. Others—vitamins and minerals—are *micronutrients*; they are a relatively small part of our diet and are not a source of energy (though some vitamins help convert calorie-containing nutrients into usable forms of energy). Even so, micronutrients are as essential to good health as their macro counterparts, and most foods contain both.

FAT-SOLUBLE OR WATER-SOLUBLE?

All vitamins are either fat-soluble or water-soluble. These categories help determine absorption, storage, and other characteristics of nutrients.

Fat-soluble vitamins are A, D, E, and K. As their name suggests, these vitamins dissolve in liquid fats but not in water. The body absorbs them through the intestinal tract membranes with the assistance of dietary fats and bile acids. Once absorbed, these vitamins are transported and stored throughout the body; in many cases the body can call upon these reserves if intake of a vitamin is low. Because these nutrients can accumulate in the body, toxic levels of vitamin A, D, and K in particular occur relatively quickly with consistently high consumption levels.

The *water-soluble* vitamins are C and all of the Bs. The body absorbs these vitamins through the gastrointestinal tract—without the help of dietary fats and bile acids—and does not store significant amounts of them. Because excess quantities are excreted (lost through urination or perspiration), the body is less likely to build up toxic levels of water-soluble vitamins than of fat-soluble vitamins. However, the fact that water-soluble vitamins are not stored means that you need to be more conscientious about consuming adequate amounts of them on a regular basis. These nutrients also tend to be less sturdy than fat-soluble nutrients and are more likely to be destroyed through cooking and when foods are stored or exposed to light for long periods of time.

GETTING STARTED WITH YOUR PERSONAL VITAMIN STRATEGY

Here is a summary of the strategies you should keep in mind as you develop your own vitamin program:

Strategy 1: The goal of vitamin intake is not just to prevent deficiency diseases, but to achieve a state of excellent health. Set your nutrient doses at a level designed to maximize well-being rather than simply to avoid symptoms associated with deficiencies.

As already noted, for decades most vitamin and mineral recommendations have been based on the lowest level necessary to prevent deficiency symptoms, with a modest margin of safety added. The scientific panel that sets the RDAs has defined its recommendations as: "…the levels of intake of essential nutrients that, on the basis of scientific knowledge, are judged by the Food and Nutrition Board to be adequate to meet the known nutrient needs of practically all healthy persons." The panel stated that it was impossible to determine and establish "optimal" doses higher than the RDAs.

This policy may be appropriate when setting standards for the population as a whole, but it is not the right answer for many individuals—for example, those who are not "healthy" (a term that is defined differently by just about everyone anyway). The RDA (and USRDA) level may be much too low for people who have medical disorders such as diabetes or kidney disease, and it is likely to be too low for large numbers of people who use alcohol or certain medications, or who have unusual dietary patterns. Some of these individuals should probably be taking dosages much larger than the RDA for some specific nutrients to compensate for their circumstances.

Also, despite what RDA panelists have said, a growing body of evidence now suggests that larger doses of at least some nutrients can do far more than simply prevent deficiency diseases, perhaps including prevention of some aging conditions once considered inevitable. To the extent you can potentially benefit from larger doses, it makes sense to increase the doses—provided the monetary cost is reasonable and the potential risk of adverse reactions is low.

One of today's assignments is to make sure you are at least reaching the vitamin USRDAs, which appear in the appendix. After reviewing all of the materials in this book about vitamins and minerals, you may wish to talk with your physician or a registered dietitian to see if higher doses of selected nutrients are appropriate in your particular case.

Strategy 2: For each nutrient, the recommended dose should provide the best balance of benefits with the least potential risk. As with most things in life, the goal of nutritional planning is to gain the greatest possible good without putting yourself in jeopardy. Whenever potential benefits of higher vitamin levels outweigh potential risks, increasing your intake of those vitamins makes sense.

As important as increased doses of particular nutrients may be, excessive amounts of some—for example, preformed vitamin A and vitamin B_6—can produce serious toxic side effects and even permanent physical damage. It's important to be prudent and cautious in using vitamin and mineral supplements, then, always trying to maximize the benefits while minimizing the risks.

In the case of vitamin E, for example, research suggests major potential benefits from larger doses, without significant risks. (No significant side effects have been found among people who have taken fairly large doses of vitamin E for long periods of time.) It may

---

RDAS, USRDAS, AND OTHER GUIDELINES

There is no shortage of vitamin and mineral recommendations. You might be most familiar with the acronym RDAs, or Recommended Dietary Allowances, which were first issued in the 1940s (by the Food and Nutrition Board of the National Academy of Science's National Research Council), and are updated periodically. However, the RDAs are somewhat complex because they incorporate separate recommendations for each sex, for different age categories (from infancy to old age), and for women who are pregnant or breast-feeding.

In the 1970s, officials at the U.S. Food and Drug Administration (FDA) felt a need to make the RDAs simpler and more accessible, particularly for placing this information on food-packaging labels. As a result, the FDA issued its own U.S. Recommended Daily Allowances, or USRDAs—a single, simplified recommendation for each vitamin and mineral. In general, the USRDAs correspond to the highest RDA for each nutrient. In this book, we'll include the USRDAs as a point of reference when making our own recommendations. (To avoid confusion between the USRDAs and RDAs, the FDA recently established the Reference Daily Intakes, or RDIs, to replace the term USRDA; RDIs have been assigned to 27 vitamins and minerals.)

To further complicate the situation, there are other guidelines and terms that you may come across. The Reference Daily Intakes are represented on nutrition labels as percent Daily Values, or DVs. Then there's the Dietary Reference Intakes, or DRIs, which are a new set of values being developed by the National Academy of Sciences to take the place of the RDAs. To date, however, the Academy has issued DRIs for only a few nutrients.

make sense then, after consulting with your physician, to boost the amount of vitamin E you consume up to our recommended dose.

The same approach applies to some of the B vitamins. Recent research has singled out homocysteine (an amino acid found in the blood) as promoting atherosclerosis and blood vessel damage. However, homocysteine levels can frequently be lowered significantly by consuming three B vitamins: folic acid, vitamin B_6 and vitamin B_{12}. For this reason (and others), doses of these vitamins above the USRDAs may provide a safe way to optimize your health, particularly if you have other risk factors for heart disease. Unfortunately, the situation is not always clear-cut.

At low doses, vitamin benefits do generally outweigh risks. But for many vitamins, few statistically sound studies have accurately measured the risks and benefits at higher intake levels. Medical literature is, however, filled with reports of dangerous side effects at extremely high doses for some nutrients. (Our own recommendations in this chapter do not reach the levels that have been reported to cause adverse side effects.)

If the risks of higher doses have not been studied, or the results of such studies are unclear, the prudent course generally is to take the lower doses until enough research has been done to demonstrate that higher levels are risk-free or that they confer sufficient additional benefits to warrant the known risks.

Strategy 3: When appropriate, personalize your strategy to meet your unique needs in terms of age, sex, size, lifestyle, and medical condition. In this chapter, you will find information about the medical conditions and lifestyle issues that can increase your need for specific nutrients.

Strategy 4: Use foods as your source of vitamins whenever possible. Through a varied and balanced diet, you can provide your body with a variety of the vitamins you need, without risks of side effects. Keep in mind, too, that foods supply you with other important substances that you cannot get from a vitamin pill, health-promoting substances ranging from energy-producing carbohydrates and proteins to cholesterol-lowering fibers.

However, it may not be possible to get all of the essential nutrients you need through foods alone, especially if your medical or lifestyle status creates an increased need for certain nutrients. If you're on a low-calorie diet for weight loss, if your body does not tolerate dairy products, or if a chronic disease interferes with your absorption of nutrients, for example, you may have to use vitamin (and mineral) supplements just to reach the minimum levels recommended for good health.

Strategy 5: Use vitamins to complement a healthful lifestyle—not to compensate for unhealthful habits. Some people believe they can make up for all kinds of undesirable behaviors by taking vitamin (and mineral) supplements. But these pills cannot replace the cardiovascular and many other benefits of exercise. And while vitamin supplements may help overcome some of the free-radical formation stimulated by cigarette smoking, they won't protect you from nicotine's destructive effects upon your heart, and they cannot protect you completely against the cancer-causing tars. If you eat large quantities of high-fat foods or have other unhealthful habits, vitamin capsules won't rescue you from a health crisis at some point in your life. Nutritional supplements should be an adjunct to the other health-enhancing behaviors that are part of your day-to-day living.

Strategy 6: Choose supplements in doses that will ensure that you'll reach the levels we recommend. As we explain in the box on page 78, there are many vitamin intake guidelines – the RDAs, the USRDAs, the RDIs, and the DRIs. Rather than trying to sort out this alphabet soup of recommendations, we have provided you with our own single recommendation of the best dose for each vitamin. By following these recommendations, you'll do more than prevent deficiencies—you'll ensure that you'll be receiving the most beneficial level of each vitamin.

HOW TO BUY VITAMINS

As you read this section, you may decide that, for the good of your health, you want to consume more vitamins than you get from your meals. Your decision may take you to the nutrient-supplement section of your supermarket, to a health food store, or to mail-order ads, where the wide array of available supplements can be boggling. But don't panic. Here are some guidelines to help you navigate through the sea of vitamin and mineral choices.

Natural or Synthetic

As you browse the vitamin shelves, you'll face a decision between *natural* and *synthetic* supplements. Natural products come from foods, while synthetic versions are manufactured in a lab. It's a confusing issue, and many consumers believe that they cheat themselves if they settle for synthetic vitamins rather than paying more for natural ones.

The truth is—despite the hype—the natural and synthetic formulations of each nutrient have the same chemical configuration, whether they were obtained from plants or made in a laboratory. Once you remove them from the bottle and swallow them, they act identically; your body won't know the difference. Some "natural" products, in fact, might actually be a combination of a little bit of plant extract and synthetic vitamins; the word *natural* means whatever the manufacturer wants it to mean.

There are exceptions to this rule: The natural and synthetic formulations of vitamin E and beta carotene have minor differences in their chemical configuration. Some people believe the natural versions have greater efficacy. Many experts disagree, saying that the variations are too subtle to be significant, but the issue is still unsettled.

Be aware, too, that some manufacturers promote their products as originating from various sources—most commonly, vitamin C from "rose hips." In general, you do not need to be concerned about these distinctions. Many "rose hip" vitamins are probably mostly synthetic, with only a small amount of the C coming from the fleshy base (the hip) of the rose itself. The rest has been manufactured in a test tube, like any other synthetic vitamin.

In addition to the natural-synthetic debate, manufacturers of some synthetic forms of vitamins (and minerals) claim that their supplements are more "available" to the body. "Ester C" for example, may have 10 percent greater "bioavailability" than traditional vitamin C. Even a 10 percent variation, however, won't make a lot of difference when you're already consuming 250 to 500 mg of vitamin C.

Where To Shop

There's no shortage of places to buy nutritional supplements. Supermarkets sell them, as do pharmacies, health food stores, some department stores, and mail-order houses. So where should you shop? Except for some variations in price, you may not find much difference among the supplements from one store to another. Only a limited number of companies manufacture vitamins and minerals. These supply brand-name products to outlets throughout the country and also repackage their items with store-brand labels. So while the names on the labels may change, the products are generally identical. Still, it's a good idea to buy supplements at a store known for selling quality merchandise.

Supplement Labels

As with any other product you buy, you should do some comparison shopping—and not only for price. Read the labels on supplements, and see what you get for your dollar. Don't allow gimmicky names—such as *stress vitamins, therapeutic formulas,* or *super vitamins*—to sway you. Instead, look at the description of what's inside the bottle, specifically at the nutrients and their potencies.

Using your personalized program as a guide, you need to determine if a multivitamin formulation can give you the amounts of each nutrient that you want. Would you be better off purchasing certain vitamin or mineral supplements individually? For most people, the answer is probably to combine a broad-spectrum multivitamin and mineral preparation with "booster" doses of selected individual nutrients to meet particular needs.

Be sure to look carefully at the quantities of nutrients in the bottle. Often you'll find quantities given in milligrams (mg), the equivalent of one-thousandth of a gram. Some vitamins and minerals are needed in such small amounts, however, that they are measured in micrograms (mcg), equal to one-millionth of a gram. Some—such as vitamins A, D, and E—may also be measured in international units (IU), designations of their biological activity, not of their weight. The labels of many products carrying IU values also provide equivalency doses in milligrams or micrograms.

When you consider price, keep in mind not only the number of tablets in the bottle, but also the amount of the nutrient in each tablet. Don't let the size of the bottle or of the capsules themselves deceive you; the quantity of a given vitamin or mineral in a single tablet can differ considerably.

The label may also give you clues about the capacity of the vitamin or mineral to dissolve in your digestive system and make its way into your bloodstream. Unless the product is a time-release formulation, it should disintegrate (break into small pieces) within an hour. If it doesn't dissolve this way—and not all pills do—it can't work in your bloodstream.

The label probably won't contain this specific information, but look for a designation that the manufacturer adheres to standards created by the US Pharmacopoeia (USP), the scientific body that sets criteria for drug composition. These guidelines require, for example, that water-soluble vitamins disintegrate in the digestive tract in no more than 30 to 45 minutes. If the label doesn't provide data about the release of the nutrients, or if it doesn't state that the product abides by USP standards, you should assume that it doesn't meet these guidelines. Also, feel free to call or write to the manufacturer and request information about the speed with which its products dissolve and disintegrate (or about any other product feature that interests you).

Check the expiration date on the label, and don't purchase a product with a date that has already passed. (If you find such a product on the store shelf, ask the manager to remove it.) If a product is within a few months of expiring—say, within six months or less—be aware that it may have already been in the bottle for a few years and lost some of its stability and potency. Look for a product that doesn't expire for a year or more.

Using Supplements

Many experts on vitamins and minerals say that your body can make use of supplements no matter what time of day you consume them. If you take them with meals, though, food can often improve the rate at which your intestines absorb the nutrients. We recommend that you take your supplements at the same time each day—perhaps with breakfast or dinner—making it a habit and reducing the chances that you'll forget to take them.

Store your supplements away from direct sunlight and heat. A cool, dry place is better than the refrigerator, where moisture can undermine the nutrients' potency.

Selecting and properly utilizing vitamin supplements takes effort. With care, though, you can maximize the benefits you get from these nutrients and place yourself on the fast track toward excellent health.

ANTIOXIDANTS

Much of the changing attitude about vitamins has come about in recent years because of a group of nutrients known as antioxidants. This group contains vitamins C and E, beta carotene (a compound that the body converts into vitamin A), and the minerals zinc and selenium. Numerous scientific journals have published studies, conducted at some of the world's most respected medical research facilities, supporting the role of these unique nutrients in preventing or ameliorating the adverse effects of major chronic diseases and illnesses, including cancer and heart disease.

How Do Antioxidants Work?

What makes antioxidants so important? Can they really help us move from ordinary to excellent health? To understand how antioxidants can help you, step back for a moment to look at your body as a whole and at its interrelationship with the environment around you.

Your body is a complex structure with several dynamic organ systems that function independently and interdependently. To sustain you in your environment, these interconnected systems require fuel. That fuel—the food you take in when you eat—is broken down into macronutrients: fats, carbohydrates, and proteins. As you read earlier, macronutrients provide the energy that enables your lungs to take in air and your heart to continuously pump blood through your body. This energy allows your brain to function, your muscles to contract, and your immune system to fight off infection.

Your body's process of consuming and using energy is called its *metabolism*. This process goes on constantly, day and night, within your body. In a way, this use of energy can be compared to a car's burning of gasoline. To run at full efficiency, the car requires not only gasoline as its energy source, but also the right additives to keep the engine from "knocking." Your body requires not only carbohydrates, protein, and fat for energy, but also the right balance of macronutrients to run at its best.

The Role Of Oxygen

Without oxygen, your body could not convert the food that you consume into usable energy. This essential substance allows you to metabolize fats, proteins, and carbohydrates. The body's use of oxygen involves a process known as oxidative reactions. These essential reactions convert food energy sources into useful molecular subunits and discard what is no longer needed or functional.

Everything you do—from the most basic actions of seeing, hearing, smelling, and tasting to the more complex activities of walking, running, laughing, sleeping, and thinking—depends on your body's use of oxygen. Oxygen is key to your survival and to the proper functioning of your vital organs.

Free Radicals

In a car, the running motor creates an exhaust that is emitted through the tailpipe. The gases in that exhaust (carbon monoxide, sulfur, and nitrogen oxides) are harmful pollutants. In a similar way, as your body uses molecules to create energy, it produces an "exhaust" that includes substances known as free radicals. Because of their structure, free radicals are toxic; you can think of them as harmful pollutants. Of the many kinds of free radicals, the most common are oxygen-free radicals. As the cells in your body consume millions of oxygen molecules each minute, huge numbers of these oxygen-free radicals are produced.

Free radicals are molecules with one or more unpaired electrons; they are unstable and highly reactive. To regain stability, free radicals attack other molecules in search of an electron. Free radicals can target molecules in any cell in the body from which to grab an electron. The molecule attacked by the free radical loses an electron and is damaged.

Just as your body constantly consumes and uses energy, the free radicals produced during this process constantly damage molecules in cells throughout your body. In fact, it is estimated that every cell in your body is subjected to approximately 10,000 "hits" by free radicals each day.

While normal metabolism produces some free radicals, many circumstances—such as illness, cigarette smoking, radiation, and irritating chemicals in the air—can increase the number of free radicals produced. When the level of free radicals gets too high, as in smokers, for example, the body is said to be in a state of oxidative stress.

Fortunately, your cells have built-in systems to repair the damage free radicals cause, and your body can usually maintain a reasonable balance between the rate of damage and the rate of repair. Under conditions of oxidative stress, however, more time may be required to repair a cell. The cell may not be damaged enough to be considered "sick," but will not function well enough to be considered healthy.

Consider, for example, the oxidative damage and repair that takes place in your body if you exercise too vigorously. The working muscles consume large quantities of oxygen and produce huge numbers of free radicals. The next day, you feel muscle fatigue, largely the effect of free radical damage. If you rest for a day or two, your muscles repair themselves and the pain goes away. This process of damage and repair is known as oxidative stress and cellular healing.

On the other hand, the damage from free radicals is sometimes too extensive to repair. If free radicals attack and damage enough molecules, cell death may occur, and entire organs may be damaged and even cease to work, or your body's DNA molecules may be permanently damaged, which could eventually trigger the development of a disease such as cancer. Some scientists believe that free radicals are responsible for or contribute significantly to the development of a number of chronic illnesses and to aging itself.

If free radicals are so bad, you may wonder, why does your body continue to produce them? Like oxygen itself—which is essential but which can be toxic—free radicals help protect your body in some important ways. Certain immune cells in your body release free radicals that can kill invading bacteria and help prevent infections, for example. Because of this, we need to balance the destructive and the beneficial capabilities of these molecules. In most cases, fortunately, you can maintain this balance through cellular repair systems and through antioxidants, substances that "neutralize" free radicals before enough of them accumulate to damage the healthy cells in your body.

Antioxidant Vitamins/Minerals

The substances that neutralize free radicals are called antioxidants. Some antioxidants occur naturally in the environment; your body manufactures others (for example, enzymes with names like *superoxide dismutase, glutathione peroxidase,* and *catalase*). As we mentioned, certain vitamins and minerals have antioxidant effects, particularly vitamins C and E, and beta carotene, as well as the minerals zinc and selenium.

Currently, our knowledge is greatest about the antioxidant effects of vitamins C and E and of beta carotene. These three micronutrients are found in different parts of the cell; which nutrient is active depends on where a free radical attacks. For example, vitamin E is fat-soluble (dissolves in fat) and is found primarily in cell membranes; it may act most prominently as an antioxidant if damage occurs in the cell membrane. The water-soluble vitamin C is found in the cytoplasm of the cell and may play a more important antioxidant role if a free radical is inside the watery confines of the cell.

Despite their different locations in the cell, antioxidants operate in similar ways. When they encounter a free radical, with its unpaired or missing electron, they give up one of their own electrons to the free radical. Once its electron is paired, the free radical is "quenched"—that is, it is no longer reactive or toxic.

Why doesn't the vitamin itself become a free radical? It does, in fact, but its structure is much more stable, so it is neither toxic nor reactive. Interestingly, antioxidants have been found to interact with each other. When vitamin E gives up its electron to a free radical, the vitamin becomes oxidized. Vitamin C can then interact with the modified vitamin E and return it to its original state. This vitamin interaction helps maintain the balance between free radicals and antioxidants.

In summation, our bodies break down the food that we consume into the nutrients that supply energy. This energy fuels the many cellular functions necessary to sustain life. Metabolism—the process of energy consumption and utilization—involves a series of reactions using oxygen. These oxidative reactions create byproducts, known as free radicals, which are highly reactive, toxic molecules with unpaired electrons. In some cases, free radicals defend the body against infections; in others, they cause cellular damage. Substances known as antioxidants help the body cope with this potential for cellular damage. Antioxidants, more notably vitamins C and E and beta carotene, give up electrons to render free radicals harmless.

ANTIOXIDANTS AND CHRONIC DISEASES

As noted earlier, some scientists believe that free radicals contribute to the development of some important medical problems and chronic diseases, including cardiovascular disease (heart disease and stroke), cancer, and cataracts. To appreciate how antioxidants may prevent or delay disease, it's important to explore the role of free radicals in these areas.

Cardiovascular Disease Due To Atherosclerosis

The primary cause of cardiovascular disease (coronary heart disease, heart attack, angina, and stroke) is a disorder called atherosclerosis, in which fat deposits, called plaque, build up in the walls of arteries. This buildup ultimately causes the openings inside the arteries to narrow, choking off the flow of blood and oxygen. If too much plaque builds up, the lack of oxygen eventually damages the organs served by the arteries. When blood flow to the heart is cut off, a heart attack occurs; when the brain is affected, a stroke results.

The process of accumulating plaque is complex and involves many factors, including elevated cholesterol levels, high blood pressure, and cigarette smoking. The level of cholesterol in the blood is important, but the action of free radicals on LDL (the so-called "bad" cholesterol) also appears to be critical. Research shows that LDL cholesterol undergoes oxidative modification when attacked by free radicals. Many experts believe that this modification accelerates plaque buildup in the arteries. This may help to explain why cigarette smokers—who have much higher levels of free radicals than nonsmokers— are more prone to suffer heart attacks.

Many laboratory studies have shown that adding vitamin E to plasma helps LDL cholesterol to resist oxidation. Recent research suggests that this effect of vitamin E (and, perhaps, the other antioxidants) may help prevent coronary heart disease in humans. Of thousands of people studied worldwide, those who consumed more antioxidants, either dietary or supplementary, were less likely to develop heart disease.

Still, it's important to keep in mind that antioxidants sometimes can have a downside, particularly when taken simultaneously with prescription drugs. One notable example emerged in a study published in 2001, whose researchers warned that if you're taking a statin drug and niacin to manage your cholesterol level, you need to be careful with the effects that antioxidants (vitamins E and C, beta carotene, selenium) may also have. They reported that when these four antioxidants were given to cardiovascular-disease patients who were also taking both simvastatin (Zocor) and niacin, the antioxidants tended to blunt the positive effects of statin therapy. The increases in good (HDL) cholesterol levels were not as high in the subjects taking antioxidants plus the drugs, compared to those taking the drugs alone.

Cancer

The other major disease linked to damage from free radicals is cancer. While we do not completely understand the mechanism involved, many scientists believe that high levels of free radicals play a role in transforming healthy cells into cancer cells. Free radicals may be involved in the development of cancers related to cigarette smoking, radiation, and chemical and physical carcinogens (such as asbestos). Some experts think that these cancers result from oxidative damage to DNA within the cells, resulting in mutations that perpetuate the production of abnormal DNA. Oxidative damage may be the first step in what is known to be a long, multistage progression from initial mutation to malignant cell.

Antioxidants seem to help most in cancers linked to free radical damage—especially those cancers involving the gastrointestinal tract (colon, stomach, esophagus, and oropharynx) and the lungs. Many studies show that antioxidants can block this kind of DNA damage. Even after damage has occurred, antioxidants may be able to reverse some of the changes, or at least halt the long progression from simple DNA damage to development of cancer (although it is unlikely that the process can be stopped or reversed by antioxidants once an actual cancer has developed).

Cataracts

Antioxidants may play an important role in preventing cataracts. Proteins, called *crystallins*, give the lens of the eye its transparency, making it the only clear organ in the body. When damaged by chronic exposure to the sun's ultraviolet rays (a potent generator of free radicals), the crystallins clump. This makes the lens opaque and causes blurred vision. The opaque area is the cataract.

A number of studies have shown that increased amounts of dietary or supplementary antioxidants can reduce the risk of developing cataracts, and research in this area is ongoing. Since cataract operations are the most common surgical procedure performed in the United States, this finding could have important economic implications. It could also provide tremendous relief from personal stress and inconvenience.

Some eye specialists believe that antioxidants may help prevent an even more serious eye disorder called age-related macular degeneration (AMD), which causes severe visual impairment and can lead to permanent blindness. Years of free radical damage may be partly responsible for this condition, which affects up to 30 percent of the people in the

United States ages 65 years and older. If free radicals are involved, antioxidants may play a protective role.

In 2001, the National Eye Institute issued an advisory statement, noting that high levels of antioxidants can significantly lower the risk of advanced AMD. In high-risk patients, high-dose combinations of vitamins C, E, beta carotene and zinc can significantly reduce the likelihood of developing this eye disorder by about 25 percent.

Aging and Depressed Immune Function

In the mid-1950s, Dr. Denham Harman suggested that free radical reactions throughout life could cause the cumulative damage and deficits often associated with aging. Now that we have the technological ability to measure free radical damage and the effects of antioxidants on free radicals, more physicians are beginning to accept the possibility that Dr. Harman's theory may be correct. Unfortunately, the government's RDAs are not always sensitive to aging concerns. Some guidelines, for instance, give one RDA for adults up to the age of 50 and another for those 51 and older. Clearly, dividing people into just two groups is a vast oversimplification. A person who is 51 years old has very different nutritional needs than someone who is 91.

Many laboratory experiments have linked free radicals to the age-related decline in immune function. Free radicals stimulate the body to produce and release larger amounts of prostaglandins, substances that can hamper some immune responses, particularly to infection. Studies show that vitamin E can reduce levels of prostaglandins. Some scientists believe that vitamin E accomplishes this by "neutralizing" free radicals.

Immune function usually appears to decline with age, but antioxidants may slow the rate of decline or even reverse it. In fact, many of the conditions we associate with aging may not be entirely related to aging.

The Future

With improving technology and expanding scientific information, researchers are looking to see if free radicals are causing or influencing a wider array of chronic diseases, and if antioxidants could prevent or ameliorate them. Among the diseases being studied are diabetes, Parkinson's disease, and Lou Gehrig's disease. Other studies, on free radicals in relation to exercise-related muscle injuries and the impact of antioxidants on recovery, may bring insights that will help maintain muscle function not only for athletes, but for the aging population.

Some recent research actually raises more questions rather than providing definitive answers. For example, in 1996, based on two rigorously controlled studies, experts at the National Cancer Institute advised that supplements of beta carotene may provide no protection against cancer and heart disease. Other scientists disagree, however. As the research continues, our own recommendations are based on the latest scientific evidence now available.

As we improve our understanding of the role of free radicals in developing chronic diseases, and as we increase our knowledge of how micronutrients like vitamins E and C and beta carotene can contribute to health, we can provide even more specific, targeted recommendations for dietary intakes.

DR. ART ULENE'S DAILY VITAMIN RECOMMENDATIONS

Vitamin A	5000 IU
Beta carotene	6–15 mg
Vitamin B_3 (niacin)	20 mg
Vitamin B_6 (pyridoxine)	4 mg
Vitamin B_{12} (cobalamin)	100 mcg
Vitamin B_1 (thiamin)	1.5–10 mg
Vitamin B_2 (riboflavin)	2–5 mg
Vitamin B_5 (pantothenic acid)	10–100 mg
Biotin	300 mcg
Vitamin C	250–500 mg
Vitamin D	400 IU
Vitamin E	200–400 IU
Folic acid	400 mcg
Vitamin K	120 mcg

DAY **9** ASSIGNMENTS

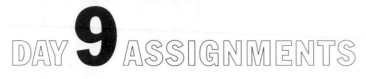

● MET GOAL ◑ PARTIALLY MET GOAL ○ MISSED GOAL

PHYSICAL VITALITY

○ 1. Improve your time for the measured mile by 2 seconds.   **Time:_____**

○ 2. Do all the flexibility and stretching exercises.

○ 3. Do leg and abdominal strength training exercises.

NUTRITIONAL VITALITY

○ 4. Decrease total fat intake to 10% of total calories.

○ 5. Eat at least 7 half-cup portions of fruits and vegetables.

○ 6. Supplement as necessary to reach the vitamin & mineral recommendations.

MENTAL VITALITY

○ 7. Spend at least 10 minutes practicing any deep relaxation technique.

○ 8. Identify and eliminate as many sources of stress in your life as you can.

EMOTIONAL & SPIRITUAL VITALITY

MEDICAL VITALITY

MINERALS

DAY 9

Minerals are inorganic substances that originate in soil and water, but find their way into the animals and plants that make up our diet. Although vitamins have received much more attention, an adequate intake of minerals is just as important to your health. Minerals play a critical role in the enzyme systems that allow biochemical reactions to occur within your body. Without adequate levels of essential minerals, your heart muscle cannot contract; oxygen cannot be carried in the red blood cells; and the development of strong bones and teeth is impossible.

Your body needs much larger quantities of many minerals than of vitamins. Each day, we need hundreds of milligrams of the minerals called macro (or major) minerals, which include calcium, sodium, potassium, chloride, phosphorus, and magnesium. Your body requires only small amounts of other minerals, called trace minerals, including iron, iodine, and copper. Relatively little is known about other trace minerals—nickel, tin, and vanadium—but researchers believe that they are probably necessary at very small levels. No one mineral is more crucial than another; your body needs all of them in appropriate quantities.

MACRO VERSUS TRACE MINERALS

Many people are quite familiar with the macro minerals, because of the publicity that many of these minerals have received in recent years. For example, as the population ages, and the risk of osteoporosis (a bone-thinning disease) affects more people, calcium has been receiving a great deal of attention in the media. The increased appreciation of the importance of calcium consumption has been accompanied by increases in the recommended dose (from a USRDA of 800 mg per day to the current level of 1,000 mg).

But while many people have become much more diligent about their need for macro minerals like calcium, the trace or micro minerals—like iron, chromium, zinc and selenium—are often overlooked, even though minute amounts of these minerals may be just as essential for the maintenance of vitality and prevention of disease. To achieve *real* vitality, you must be just as conscientious about your consumption of these micro minerals as you are about the better known major minerals.

At the same time, be aware that these minerals must be approached with a degree of caution. As with all vitamins and minerals, you can get too much of a good thing, and in very large doses, trace minerals (also called "trace elements") can become toxic. Despite claims by some supplement proponents that large doses of these micronutrients can cure all kinds of health problems, the evidence is scarce and the dangers are real.

For example, some studies have suggested that an excessive intake of iron might be linked to an increased risk of coronary heart disease. More recent research has raised doubts about this possible association (one study even showed that iron has a protective effect against heart disease), but the issue is still not settled. Until we know more, iron is a good example of a micro mineral that, while important, should not be consumed in excess.

Keep in mind that your body maintains a delicate balance of chemicals and nutrients, which can be undermined by overrelying on any single substance. In fact, the concept of "megadoses" has no place when you're talking about trace minerals. If you use supplements of any mineral, read the labels carefully, and talk to your doctor before consuming higher levels than are recommended on the label.

Concerns about toxicity have driven some people in the other direction with respect to consumption of both macro and micro minerals. They worry that over time, even modest amounts of minerals will accumulate in the body, causing adverse effects. This concern is unfounded if you are consuming trace minerals in foods and supplementing at recommended levels, except in a very small number of people who have congenital disorders that cause abnormal storage of certain minerals.

WHAT YOU NEED TO KNOW

Much of what you've already read about vitamins in Day 8 also applies to minerals, from the natural-versus-synthetic supplement debate, to the best way to take these pills. As with vitamins, your goal with minerals is to use them not just to prevent deficiency diseases (although prevention is very important), but also to achieve optimal health.

As a first step, you need to be sure that you're meeting the U.S. Recommended Daily Allowance (USRDA) for each mineral. But, keep in mind that these recommended doses are the *minimum* amounts necessary for healthy people to prevent deficiency disorders. Some nutritional experts believe that—at least for some of the minerals—the USRDAs may not be the best amounts to consume, especially for people with medical conditions that increase the need for particular minerals.

This program will help you identify your particular needs for each of the essential minerals. For some of these minerals, you will find that our recommended intake exceeds the USRDA. We have recommended higher levels only when there is evidence that the overall potential benefits of these higher doses outweigh the overall risks. Be aware, however, that some individuals may not be able to tolerate these higher doses. Before taking any dose that exceeds a USRDA, you should talk first with your physician to be sure that the larger dose is appropriate in your particular case. (As you'll see, in the case of iron, our recommendation may actually be a little *lower* than the USRDA for some individuals for reasons explained in the appendix.)

FOOD FIRST

As with vitamins, minerals should be obtained first and foremost from your diet. You should be able to reach the USRDAs for most minerals simply by eating a wide variety of foods regularly. Good eating habits will also help you acquire many other natural health-promoting substances that are found in foods—above and beyond simple vitamins and minerals.

It is not difficult to meet the USRDAs for most minerals if you are eating a balanced diet with a wide variety of foods. If you are unable to reach the USRDAs with diet alone, you should give serious consideration to mineral supplementation. If you choose to take supplements, your physician, dietitian or pharmacist can help you select an appropriate product.

In the appendix, you will find a great deal of useful information about several minerals that are essential for health. By reviewing this material, you will become familiar with the unique features of each mineral. You'll also find our recommendations for your intake of these minerals, which appear below as well.

DR. ART ULENE'S DAILY MINERAL RECOMMENDATIONS	
Calcium	1,500 mg
Iron	10 mg for men
	15 mg for women who are menstruating
	(up to 20 mg for women with heavy menstrual bleeding)
	10 mg for women after menopause
Magnesium	500 mg
Selenium	200 mcg
Zinc	15 mg

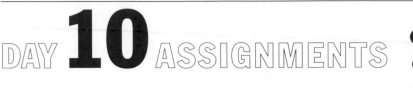

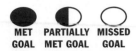

MET GOAL   PARTIALLY MET GOAL   MISSED GOAL

PHYSICAL VITALITY

1. Improve your time for the measured mile by 2 seconds.   **Time**:_____
2. Do all the flexibility and stretching exercises.

NUTRITIONAL VITALITY

3. Decrease total fat intake to 10% of total calories.
4. Eat at least 7 half-cup portions of fruits and vegetables.
5. Supplement as necessary to reach the vitamin & mineral recommendations.
6. Limit dietary cholesterol to 300 mg per day.

MENTAL VITALITY

7. Spend at least 10 minutes practicing any deep relaxation technique.
8. Identify and eliminate as many sources of stress in your life as you can.

EMOTIONAL & SPIRITUAL VITALITY

MEDICAL VITALITY

CHOLESTEROL   DAY 10

Cholesterol is a waxy, odorless substance that is found in foods of animal origin, including beef, poultry, fish, cheese, eggs, and dairy products. In general, the more cholesterol you put into your body by eating such foods, the higher your blood cholesterol concentration will be. But dietary cholesterol is not the only determinant of your blood cholesterol level. The amount of fat (especially saturated fat) you eat, and the amount of cholesterol your liver manufactures on its own, also play important roles.

The body requires some cholesterol for good health. Cholesterol is used to build the walls of cells throughout your body and to manufacture other essential substances, like hormones and vitamin D; in very young children, cholesterol plays an important role in the development of the brain. So it's important to have some cholesterol circulating throughout the bloodstream at all times.

It is only when the amount of cholesterol in the blood becomes too high that health hazards begin to appear. By damaging your arteries and increasing your risk of coronary heart disease, an elevated cholesterol level can keep you from achieving *real* vitality.

THE ROLE OF LIPOPROTEINS

Pure cholesterol can't mix with or dissolve in solutions like water and blood, so it is combined in your liver with other substances (fats and proteins) to form particles that are capable of moving through the bloodstream. These particles, called lipoproteins, carry cholesterol from the liver to all parts of the body where it is needed, and then bring it back again for removal from the body. There are different types of lipoproteins, including:

Very low density lipoproteins (VLDLs, or VLDL cholesterol)

Low density lipoproteins (LDLs, or LDL cholesterol)

High density lipoproteins (HDLs, or HDL cholesterol)

Each of these cholesterol forms can be measured separately in your blood. Together they make up your "total blood cholesterol" or "total cholesterol."

Very Low Density Lipoproteins (VLDLs)

The liver combines cholesterol, proteins, and fats (including triglycerides, which are blood fats) to form very low density lipoproteins, or VLDLs. These particles derive their name from the relatively low weight or density of their protein. As these VLDLs travel throughout the body, most of the triglycerides are removed, either for energy or to be stored as fat. In the process, the VLDLs are eventually converted to LDLs, which are described below.

Low Density Lipoproteins (LDLs)

Once triglycerides are removed from the VLDLs, the smaller particles that remain contain mostly cholesterol and protein. These particles are called low density lipoproteins, or LDLs. Many of these LDLs are removed from the bloodstream by cells throughout the body; in the cells, they are broken down into their original elements and used for essential bodily functions. However, this process does not always progress smoothly. Some people's systems remove LDLs more slowly than others, and this causes the level of LDLs (and, therefore, the level of cholesterol) to build up in their blood. (This tendency to remove LDLs and cholesterol quickly or slowly is inherited.)

If the blood level of LDL cholesterol becomes too high, there is a tendency for the cholesterol and other fatty substances to deposit in the walls of arteries. This process, known as atherosclerosis, gradually narrows the arteries and chokes off the flow of blood through them. This is the reason why LDLs have gained the nickname "bad" cholesterol— they are the real culprit in the development of coronary heart disease that is due to high blood cholesterol. When doctors talk about getting your blood cholesterol level down, they are really concerned about decreasing the LDL portion of it.

In most people, about 60 to 70 percent of all the cholesterol in the blood is in the form of LDLs, so if your LDL cholesterol level is very high, your total blood cholesterol level is likely to be high, too. Also, if your LDL level goes up or down significantly, your total blood cholesterol level will tend to rise or fall significantly. That is why the less expensive measurement of "total cholesterol" is often used to screen people for cholesterol problems and to monitor people who are trying to lower their levels.

High Density Lipoproteins (HDLs)

Though high density lipoproteins also contain some cholesterol combined with proteins and fats, these particles have a very different effect within the body. HDLs act as scavengers or "biological vacuum cleaners" within the bloodstream, attracting cholesterol and carrying it back to the liver. There, it is either reprocessed into new VLDL particles, or broken down into substances called bile acids and removed from the body. HDLs actually help to *reduce* the amount of cholesterol that is present in the blood and available to damage arteries. For that reason, HDL cholesterol has been nicknamed "good" cholesterol. The higher your HDL level, the less risk you will generally have of developing coronary heart disease.

WHAT IS YOUR RISK?

The likelihood that a person will develop coronary heart disease (narrowing down and blockage of the arteries that supply blood to the heart muscle) is directly related to the amount of cholesterol he or she has in the blood. The higher the level of blood cholesterol, the greater the risk of coronary heart disease. Cholesterol *does* count.

It was once thought that the amount of cholesterol in your blood had to rise above a certain level (the so-called "risk threshold") before your risk of heart disease started to go up. As recently as the late 1970s, many scientists and physicians insisted that your blood cholesterol level was not abnormal until it exceeded 300, because they believed that the risk of heart disease was not increased until that level was reached.

Newer studies show that the risk of a heart attack actually begins to rise as the total blood cholesterol level passes 140 to 150, and continues to increase as the cholesterol level goes up. The Framingham Heart Study, probably the best-known study of heart disease in

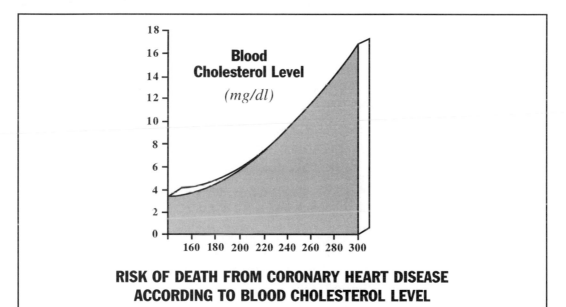

RISK OF DEATH FROM CORONARY HEART DISEASE
ACCORDING TO BLOOD CHOLESTEROL LEVEL

This chart is based on a study of 361,662 men ages 35 to 57 who were followed for an average of about six years. The figures on the left represent the number of men per thousand who died from coronary heart disease during the six-year period. For example, among men whose cholesterol levels were 180, four per thousand died. Approximately seven per thousand died among men whose cholesterol levels were 220. Notice that the risk of dying from a heart attack increases continuously as the blood cholesterol level rises. The pace at which the risk increases begins to accelerate after the cholesterol level passes 200.

the United States, examined this issue in depth. Researchers have kept constant track of the health of nearly the entire population of Framingham, Massachusetts, since 1948. They found that the risk of a heart attack begins to rise gradually when the blood cholesterol level hits the 150 level and then increases more steeply after the level exceeds 200. The study reveals that an individual whose total blood cholesterol level is 300 has about four times the risk of coronary heart disease than a person whose level is 200. Though the risk is quite small below 150, Framingham's researchers concluded that *no* cholesterol level will guarantee that an individual is free of all risk of developing coronary heart disease.

If your blood cholesterol level is high, for each 1 percent you lower it, you can reduce your chances of coronary heart disease by about 2 percent. A 15 percent reduction of your cholesterol—from 250 to 212, for example—could lower your risk of a heart attack as much as 30 percent!

But this formula is applicable only up to a point. If you were able to reduce your cholesterol level by 50 percent (perhaps from 320 to 160), you could not expect your risk of coronary heart disease to fall 100 percent—or literally to zero. No matter how well you do in reducing your cholesterol, there's no guarantee that you'll never experience a heart attack. Even so, this two-to-one guideline is an indication of just how significant each incremental decline in your total cholesterol level can be.

HDL (or "good") cholesterol can actually lower the incidence of heart attacks. Some of the most persuasive evidence for this comes from the Framingham Heart Study. In 1986, for instance, investigators there reported on the relationship between HDL cholesterol and heart disease in men and women ages forty-nine and over. Whether an individual's total cholesterol was high or low, the risk of heart disease was cut as HDL levels rose. Those people who had high HDL concentrations (at the 80th percentile) had half the risk of heart disease as those with low concentrations (at the 20th percentile).

A 1987 scientific report added weight to the theory that the risk of heart attacks could be reduced by steps that made HDL cholesterol levels go up. Researchers with the Helsinki Heart Study published their findings involving more than 4,000 middle-aged men with elevated cholesterol levels (an average of 270). These individuals received either the cholesterol-lowering drug, gemfibrozil, or a placebo for five years. Compared to the placebo group, the individuals taking gemfibrozil experienced an average decrease of 8 percent in their total cholesterol level. Based on the two-to-one formula cited above, you would expect this 8 percent drop in cholesterol to result in a 16 percent decline in heart attacks. But, in fact, the results were much more impressive. The incidence of coronary heart disease was 34 percent lower in the drug group. At the same time, the death rate from coronary heart disease was 26 percent lower.

Why were these declines in heart attacks so high? Researchers believe that increases in HDL (of about 10 percent) and/or decreases in blood triglycerides in these men probably deserve the credit. In other words, even these moderate improvements in HDL cholesterol appeared to play an important role in slashing heart-attack risks.

Even more startling were the results of a study published in 1987, which revealed that it may be possible to *reverse* atherosclerotic blockage of the arteries by reducing the blood cholesterol level. Just ten years earlier, most scientists would have scoffed at the suggestion that hardening of the arteries due to cholesterol deposits could be reversed, but Dr. David Blankenhorn and his colleagues at the University of Southern California decided to test this notion. They recruited a group of 162 men ages 40 to 59 who had previously undergone coronary bypass surgery. Angiograms were performed to confirm that these men had blockage in their arteries, and the researchers measured the exact size of the openings that remained in the blood vessels. Half of the subjects were placed on a strict low-fat, low-cholesterol diet and cholesterol-lowering drugs (colestipol and niacin). The other half were given a less restricted low-fat diet and a placebo instead of drugs.

ABOUT TRIGLYCERIDES

Triglycerides are a type of fatty substance that your doctor may talk about as you work together on your cholesterol-lowering program. Blood triglyceride levels tend to be elevated in people who have high cholesterol levels, in people with diabetes or chronic kidney disease, and in those who are obese.

The relationship between triglycerides and coronary heart disease is still controversial. Although some studies suggest that high blood triglyceride levels might increase the risk of coronary heart disease, other research fails to substantiate this association. However, there does appear to be a link between high triglycerides, low HDL levels, and forms of LDL that are particularly prone to form plaques on arterial walls.

If your blood triglyceride level is markedly elevated, your physician may recommend therapy designed to lower it. This can be accomplished by dietary change, exercise, and weight loss in most people. The use of medication to lower triglycerides while improving HDL and LDL readings may be necessary in some cases. The issue of triglycerides is complicated, however, because levels can become so variable, changing as much as 100 points from one measurement to the next. Stress, diet, and physical activity can greatly influence a particular trigylceride reading. For example, if an individual has not fasted for 9 to 12 hours before testing, the measurement may not be reliable.

The 2001 revisions of the National Cholesterol Education Program, which include triglyceride classifications, appear on page 107.

The results: The drug-treated men experienced an average 26 percent drop in their total blood cholesterol (from 246 to 180), compared to 4 percent in the other group. Perhaps even more significantly, repeat angiograms taken after the two-year study revealed that blockages in the coronary arteries had actually *regressed* in 16 percent of the men on the strict diet and drug regimen. In another 45 percent, the lesions were unchanged, indicating that the deterioration process had been halted. Even in the men receiving the low-fat diet without drugs, 37 percent had unchanged lesions, and about 2 percent showed a regression. In this placebo group, the lower the fat content in the diet, the better. While those volunteers who ate a higher-fat diet (34 percent of calories from fat) tended to develop new fatty deposits, those consuming a lower-fat diet (28 percent of calories from fat) tended to have no progression of the blockages in their arteries. The proof was there: Atherosclerosis *could* be halted and, in some cases, reversed.

Incidentally, while reading the studies cited above, you may have noticed that cholesterol-lowering drugs were often used to achieve the major improvements in cholesterol levels. In most of these large studies, the participants were individuals with very high cholesterol levels, and researchers gave drugs to some of them as one means of dealing with their condition. But there is every reason to believe that the same positive changes can be achieved *without* medications. Dr. Dean Ornish at the University of California at San Francisco School of Medicine has conducted some of the most impressive research demonstrating that lifestyle changes alone can reverse heart disease. In one study (also mentioned in Day 1), a group of Dr. Ornish's heart disease patients made significant changes in their diet and lifestyle, including adopting a very low-fat vegetarian diet, in which only 10 percent of calories came from fat. They ate no animal products except for egg whites and a cup of skim milk or yogurt per day. They also participated in a stress reduction program and moderate exercise, and they stopped smoking. Another group of patients—the "control" group—was instructed not to make changes in their lifestyle, and maintained a diet in which they consumed about 30 percent of their calories from dietary fat.

A year later, angiograms showed that 82 percent of the treatment group experienced changes toward reversal of the blockages in their coronary arteries, along with a decline in total cholesterol of 24 percent. By comparison, 53 percent of those in the control group showed progression, or worsening, of their disease.

WHAT DETERMINES YOUR TOTAL CHOLESTEROL LEVEL?

Everyone, then, has some cholesterol in the bloodstream—that's a desirable situation. What we're concerned about is *excess* cholesterol—a condition that can be caused by several different factors. Although some of these causes are beyond your control, most are quite manageable, providing you with different ways you can influence your own cholesterol level. Let's look at the factors that determine your blood cholesterol level.

Intrinsic Factors

Intrinsic factors are those that are "built into" your body makeup and therefore tend to be out of your direct control. They include heredity, age, and sex. Heredity plays perhaps the most important role, by determining how rapidly LDL cholesterol is removed from your bloodstream and how much new cholesterol is manufactured by your liver.

Even if there is no cholesterol in the foods you eat, your liver should produce as much cholesterol as your body needs for good health. However, some people inherit a tendency to overproduce cholesterol. Their livers produce *much* more than their bodies could ever utilize, and their total cholesterol levels reach 400, 500, or even more. Such high levels predispose people to the development of atherosclerosis at a very young age and to the occurrence of heart attacks as early as their thirties and forties. This type of cholesterol problem runs in families, so if your mother or father had an extremely high cholesterol level, you may have inherited the tendency.

Another intrinsic factor that influences your blood cholesterol level is your age. As you grow older, your total blood cholesterol level will tend naturally to rise. As a result, a seventy-year-old man with a cholesterol count of 215 may not have nearly as much to worry about as a thirty-five-year-old man with the same reading.

Your sex is also an influence upon your susceptibility to heart disease. The male sex is much more at risk than females; particularly before menopause, women are less vulnerable to a heart attack. Studies show that women tend to have higher HDL ("good") cholesterol levels than men of the same age. However, this natural advantage of women can be overshadowed by other factors, such as the use of oral contraceptives. Some types of birth control pills may raise the total cholesterol level slightly, while lowering the HDL cholesterol count—both undesirable consequences. The effect that oral contraceptives have on cholesterol can vary considerably, depending on the proportions of estrogen and progesterone in the pills. (It may differ from one brand to another.) If you are using birth control pills and you have high blood cholesterol, your doctor may want to measure your cholesterol level more frequently to monitor this potential effect.

Even though you can't change your heredity, your age, or your sex, you *can* compensate for any problems they cause by making a real effort to manage those factors that are subject to your control. Let's take a look at these influences.

Intake Factors

Intake factors are those related to the food you eat. They are extremely important for most people with cholesterol problems because they usually have a significant effect on the blood cholesterol level and because they can easily be controlled. The most important intake factors are saturated fats and dietary cholesterol—in that order.

Dietary Fats

Biochemists classify fats into three major categories—saturated, polyunsaturated, and monounsaturated—based on a certain characteristic of their chemical structure.

Saturated fats are found primarily in animal products, particularly fatty meats (beef, veal, lamb, pork, ham) and many dairy items (whole milk, cream, ice cream, cheese). For example, the marbleized fat you can see on beef is saturated. Some types of vegetable products—coconut oil, palm oil, palm kernel oil, and vegetable shortening—are also high in saturates. Because they are inexpensive and taste good, these highly saturated vegetable fats are frequently used in commercially baked goods and snack foods such as cookies and crackers.

These foods rich in saturated fat should be kept to a minimum in your diet. The liver uses saturated fats to manufacture cholesterol. Therefore, excessive dietary intake of saturated fats can significantly raise the blood cholesterol, especially in people who have inherited a tendency toward high blood cholesterol. Guidelines issued by the National Cholesterol Education Program and widely supported by most experts recommend that your intake of saturated fats should be less than 10 percent of your total calorie intake. However, for people who have severe problems with high blood cholesterol, even that level may be too high.

Polyunsaturated fats, on the other hand, may actually lower your total blood cholesterol level. However, in doing so, large amounts of polyunsaturates have a tendency to reduce your HDL ("good") cholesterol level, so it makes no sense to overdo your intake of this kind of fat. Several vegetable oils are rich in polyunsaturated fats, particularly corn, soybean, safflower, and sunflower seed oil, as well as certain fish oils (particularly the omega-3 fatty acids found in cold-water marine fish, such as cod, halibut and tuna). Monounsaturated fats appear to modestly reduce blood levels of LDL cholesterol without affecting HDL in any way. Monounsaturated fats are found in oils—especially olive and peanut oils—and are also prevalent in some margarines.

One other element could become an important factor in the cholesterol equation. Recent research into *trans fatty acids* suggests that they, too, might play a detrimental role in blood cholesterol levels. Trans fatty acids are fats that have been manipulated molecularly into new configurations in the laboratory, often as a way to harden liquid vegetable oils for use in foods like margarine and shortening. Trans fats are also common in packaged baked goods (cookies, crackers, doughnuts) and restaurant fried foods, and they make up 4 to 7 percent of the dietary fat consumed by Americans. One recent study found that trans monounsaturated fatty acids raised LDL cholesterol levels, so that they behaved much like saturated fats; simultaneously, these same trans fatty acids reduced HDL cholesterol readings.

Much more research is still necessary, since some studies have not produced clear-cut conclusions about these trans fatty acids. But some findings are already rather ominous. In a study by researchers in the Netherlands, published in 2001, trans fats reduced the functioning of blood vessels (i.e., their ability to dilate and expand) by about one-third, and lowered HDL cholesterol levels by about one-fifth, compared to saturated fats. This suggests that trans fats pose a greater likelihood of contributing to cardiovascular disease than saturated fats.

For now, from a cholesterol-lowering point of view, polyunsaturated and monounsaturated fats are much more desirable than saturated fats and trans fats. As a general rule, the American Heart Association currently recommends that your saturated fat intake should be 7 to 10 percent of calories, polyunsaturated fats up to 10 percent, and monounsaturated fats up to 15 percent of calories. By limiting your overall consumption of fats and oils to about 5 to 8 teaspoons a day, says the AHA, you are unlikely to consume trans fatty acids in excess. (Trans fats have been called "phantom fats" because they are not required to be listed on food labels.) The AHA guidelines also recommend that you keep your total fat intake at 30 percent or below of your daily calorie intake although in our opinion, even lower is better. For more information about fats, refer to Day 1.

Dietary Cholesterol

Although saturated fat is the major dietary contributor to high blood cholesterol, the cholesterol that is present in the foods you eat also plays a significant role. As you've read, even if you ate no cholesterol, your liver would manufacture all the cholesterol your body needs. The dietary cholesterol you consume only sets you up for excess levels of cholesterol in your blood, though it is probably not as powerful an influence as the saturated fat in your diet.

There is no cholesterol in plant foods like fruits, vegetables, and cereals, but dietary cholesterol is present in many of the other foods we eat. It is found not only in animal tissues (meat, poultry, fish) but also in animal products such as milk, cheese, butter, and eggs. You do not need to avoid cholesterol entirely in order to lower your blood cholesterol level, but you do need to limit the amount you eat to less than 300 milligrams per day according to the AHA; if you have heart disease or its risk factors, limit your intake to 200 milligrams a day. (The average American consumes about 350 to 450 milligrams of cholesterol per day.)

About 70 to 80 percent of the population are sensitive to the cholesterol in their diet. The more they eat, the higher their cholesterol levels will go. The other 20 to 30 percent are less sensitive, or even insensitive, to cholesterol in their diets. Their blood cholesterol levels will not fluctuate significantly, no matter how much or how little dietary cholesterol is consumed. For these individuals, even if they were able to cut out all the cholesterol from their diets, their blood cholesterol would stay about the same.

The trouble is there's no way of knowing whether you are one of these cholesterol-resistant individuals without undergoing some exhaustive and impractical tests. If you are sensitive to cholesterol, eating too many eggs and other cholesterol-rich foods can raise the cholesterol level in your blood. If you already have high blood cholesterol readings, you should assume that excess dietary cholesterol can sabotage your health.

Cholesterol and saturated fat tend to go hand in hand—foods that are low in saturated fat also tend to be low in cholesterol, and foods that are high in one are likely to be high in the other. There are some exceptions to this general rule, and it's important to be aware of them so they don't spoil the effect of the other cholesterol-reducing efforts you are making. For example, although liver is low in saturated fat (less than 2 grams in a 3.5-ounce portion), it is extremely high in cholesterol—almost 400 milligrams of cholesterol are present in the same-size portion. Shrimp also stands out: 3.5 ounces of this shellfish contain less than 1 gram of saturated fat and almost 200 milligrams of cholesterol. Of course, the best-known high-cholesterol culprit is the egg. An average egg has less than 2 grams of saturated fat—but 213 milligrams of cholesterol. Eat just one egg, and you have filled most of your cholesterol quota for the day.

Actually, it's the egg yolk, not the white, that contains the cholesterol. So although you should limit the number of *whole* eggs you eat, there is no need to slow down your consumption of *whites*. (This part of the egg contains no cholesterol at all.) Many people discard the yolks before they cook eggs, and find—often to their surprise—that the egg whites retain much of the "eggy" flavor. Try it yourself—use just the whites to make an omelette or scrambled eggs. *Everyone* should adhere to the American Heart Association's current recommendation, which is to eat no more than three to four egg yolks per week, and keep your total daily cholesterol intake below 300 milligrams.

As you try to curtail your egg intake, keep in mind that egg yolks are used in the manufacture of many processed and cooked food products. For most people, the majority of their egg consumption comes from the "invisible" eggs that are parts of foods such as pancakes or French toast. Eggs are also often included in breads, cakes, cookies, ice cream, mayonnaise, meat loaf, pastas, puddings, quiche, and salad dressings, so these foods should be eaten in thoughtful quantities. Do your shopping carefully, too. Read the label of every product you buy at the market and you'll discover dozens of eggs that you never realized you were eating. Incidentally, commercial egg substitutes—which do not contain yolks—are acceptable alternatives to eating natural eggs. They are made almost exclusively from egg whites, along with a small amount of fat and they can be used in cooking or for egg dishes like omelettes and quiche.

In addition to egg yolks, you also should carefully control the amount of organ meat you consume. If you are one of those people who still enjoys an occasional course of liver and onions, eat it only occasionally, because a single 3.5-ounce serving will exceed your total allowance of cholesterol for the day. Other organ meats—including brain, heart, tongue, kidneys, sweetbreads (thymus), and chitterlings—fare no better, with most having between 180 and 470 milligrams of cholesterol in a 3.5-ounce serving. And if you think that chicken liver might be an acceptable alternative to beef liver, think again. Chicken liver has 631 milligrams of cholesterol per 3.5-ounce serving!

Absorption Factors

Absorption factors help to lower your blood cholesterol level by blocking absorption of substances from the intestines that the body uses to make more cholesterol. These absorption factors include a natural tool known as soluble dietary fiber, as well as prescription cholesterol-lowering medications.

Dietary fiber is found in plant foods. The soluble variety of fiber seems to have the power to *attract* certain fatty substances in the gastrointestinal tract, escorting them to the stool and out of the body; this prevents the body from using them to manufacture cholesterol in the liver, so your blood cholesterol level goes down. High fiber diets also tend to slow the rate of digestion and food absorption, and they provide a feeling of satiety or a "full" stomach.

The richest sources of fiber are vegetables, whole-grain breads and cereals, brown rice, beans and other legumes, and fruits. Within these groups, there are many specific foods that are especially high in the amount of *soluble* fiber they contain, such as kidney or pinto beans, black-eyed peas, and oat bran. That makes these foods especially effective in helping you lower your blood cholesterol level. However, many foods that would seem to be very similar to these, such as wheat bran, lettuce, and spinach, contain primarily *insoluble* fiber. Even though these foods are very high in their total amount of dietary fiber, they are not the best alternatives in their general food groups if lowering blood cholesterol levels is your goal.

Absorption factors are more important in cholesterol control than many people realize—perhaps just as significant as reducing your intake of dietary fat and cholesterol. Moderate cutbacks in fat and cholesterol, such as those recommended by the American Heart Association, will lower total cholesterol by 5-15 percent in most people. Modest additions of soluble dietary fiber are capable of creating equally large drops. Put the two strategies together, and you have a program that in many people can lower blood cholesterol levels by 20 percent or more—without any major sacrifice. For a more detailed discussion of the importance of fiber in your diet, see Day 15 (pages 137-139).

WHAT DETERMINES YOUR HDL LEVEL?

As you have already learned, not all of the cholesterol in your bloodstream is bad for you. The HDL (high density lipoprotein) cholesterol actually has a protective effect against coronary heart disease, so the higher your HDL cholesterol level, the better. A number of factors can influence the HDL level:

- *Heredity:* As with cholesterol in general, the HDL portion is influenced by heredity. If you have inherited a tendency toward a high level of HDL, you should consider yourself fortunate.

- *Exercise:* Physical activity is one of the best ways to raise your HDL level, so if you want to increase it, you ought to get your body moving. You don't need to exercise to the point of exhaustion; research shows that a program of regular, moderate activity can raise HDL levels significantly. For a discussion of the relationship between exercise and HDL cholesterol—and how to get started with exercise—refer to Day 4 (pages 55-65).

- *Smoking:* Smoking can reduce HDL levels, which is just one of the ways that cigarettes increase the risk of heart attacks. By quitting cigarettes, you can raise your HDL and decrease your chances of a heart attack.

- *Weight:* As your weight goes up, your HDL concentration tends to decline. By losing weight, you can reverse the process. In a study by University of Pennsylvania researchers, published in 1981, a group of men who lost an average of 24 pounds elevated their HDL levels by 5 percent. Though this may not sound like much compared to the percentage decreases that we have been describing for LDL cholesterol, a small increase in HDL cholesterol can make a very significant difference in the risk of heart attacks due to atherosclerosis.

HOW HIGH IS TOO HIGH FOR YOU?

As you've read, the risk of developing heart disease actually begins to rise after the blood cholesterol level exceeds about 150, but initially this increase in risk is slight. The higher the cholesterol rises, the more rapidly the cardiovascular risk increases. A cholesterol level of 200 raises the heart attack risk about 50 percent over a level of 150. But the next 50 points have a much more dramatic effect. A cholesterol level of 250 increases the heart-attack risk by about three times over the 150 figure.

Here are the current blood cholesterol and triglyceride classifications from an expert panel of the National Cholesterol Education Program, which were revised in 2001. These blood levels should be measured after a 9- to 12-hour fast.

Total Blood Cholesterol

Less than 200 mg/dl = desirable blood cholesterol

200-239 mg/dl = borderline-high blood cholesterol

240 mg/dl or more = high blood cholesterol

LDL Cholesterol

Less than 100 mg/dl = optimal LDL cholesterol

100-129 mg/dl = near optimal LDL cholesterol

130-159 mg/dl = borderline-high LDL cholesterol

160-189 mg/dl = high LDL cholesterol

190 mg/dl or more = very high LDL cholesterol

HDL Cholesterol

Less than 40 mg/dl = low HDL cholesterol

60 mg/dl or more = high HDL

Triglycerides

Less than 150 mg/dl = normal triglycerides

150-199 mg/dl = borderline-high triglycerides

200-499 mg/dl = high triglycerides

500 mg/dl or more = very high triglycerides

How did the experts arrive at these clear-cut dividing lines between "desirable," "borderline," and "high" levels? Their decision had to be somewhat arbitrary, since the risk of heart disease goes up continually as the total cholesterol and the LDL cholesterol levels rise above certain levels, but they justified these "cut-points" because they are the approximate levels at which the risk of heart disease begins to rise more steeply.

The panel recommended that all adults twenty years of age and older have a complete lipoprotein profile performed every five years. This blood test, conducted after a 12-hour fast, should measure total cholesterol, LDL cholesterol, HDL cholesterol, and triglycerides. (This new guideline reflected a change from earlier recommendations that called for evaluating only total and HDL cholesterol in the initial screenings.) Under the new recommendations, if an individual has *not* fasted, then only total cholesterol and HDL cholesterol measurements should be taken; if the total cholesterol level turns out to be too high (at or above 200 mg/dl), or the HDL cholesterol level is too low (below 40 mg/dl), then follow-up testing should be conducted to evaluate LDL cholesterol and triglyceride levels.

Depending on the outcomes of these tests—and whether you already have evidence of coronary heart disease and/or its risk factors as evaluated in a series of tables—your doctor may provide additional evaluation, guidance or treatment. This may include additional testing in the future, an exercise program, dietary changes, and modification of your risk factors. If your cholesterol remains high despite non-drug therapy, your doctor may consider drug treatment. In fact, the updated guidelines are expected to increase the number of people receiving dietary treatment from 52 million (under the old guidelines) to 65 million, while increasing the number of those on cholesterol-lowering drugs from 13 million to 36 million.

HOMOCYSTEINE—THE NEW CHOLESTEROL?

If you haven't heard about homocysteine, you probably will soon. Homocysteine is an amino acid (a building block of protein), and it occurs naturally as a by-product of the body's metabolism of protein. If you have too much homocysteine in your bloodstream, however, your risk of heart attacks and stroke may rise. In fact, many cardiologists believe that homocysteine should be categorized as an independent risk factor for heart disease. A study at the University of Washington, published in the journal *JAMA* in 1995, concluded that high homocysteine levels were responsible for 10 percent of the population's risk of coronary artery disease; an increase in plasma homocysteine of 5 mg/dl could increase coronary risks as much as a rise of 20 mg/dl of serum cholesterol levels, according to the researchers.

Although homocysteine levels can be measured, neither the government nor the American Heart Association recommends routine testing because of the high cost of the currently available tests. Nevertheless, there are some people who may benefit from being tested for homocysteine now, including those who already have coronary heart disease or those with a strong family history of CHD.

Some research indicates that in individuals with high homocysteine levels, supplementation with folic acid and perhaps vitamin B_{12} may reduce their homocysteine values. As a result, an increasing number of doctors are recommending that people begin taking multivitamins or folic acid supplements.

A healthy diet may be beneficial as well. In a study published in 2000 by researchers at Johns Hopkins Medical Institutions and other research facilities, people who adopted the so-called DASH diet to reduce their blood pressure also lowered their levels of homocysteine after eight weeks. DASH (Dietary Approaches to Stop Hypertension) is a low-fat diet that includes plenty of fruits, vegetables, and low-fat dairy products. A change to the DASH regimen, according to the investigators, lowered homocysteine levels enough to reduce the risk of heart disease by 7 to 9 percent, in addition to its benefits associated with reductions in blood pressure.

Just how effective are these cholesterol-reducing drugs? A study published in the *New England Journal of Medicine* in November 2001 found that treatment with a "statin" drug called simvastatin (Zocor) in combination with niacin (a B vitamin) lowered by 70 percent the risk of a fatal or non-fatal heart attack or hospitalization for chest pain among patients likely to experience heart attacks and death from coronary heart disease. Statin drugs are commonly used to reduce LDL cholesterol, while niacin can increase levels of HDL cholesterol. In the study group receiving both simvastatin and niacin, the average HDL level rose 26 percent, while the average LDL level declined 43 percent. The combination of the drug and the B vitamin also actually reversed the buildup of plaque in the coronary arteries.

As you use these guidelines, there are some important points to keep in mind. For instance, the term "desirable" was used to describe blood cholesterol levels up to 199; while 199 may be desirable when compared to a level of 240, it still results in a significantly higher risk of coronary heart disease than does a level of 160. The fact is, most Americans with blood cholesterol levels of 190 could easily reduce their levels to 160 or lower, simply by changing their diets. That would significantly lower their risk of subsequent heart attacks. So don't let the "desirable" label discourage you from making changes that can reduce your cholesterol level even further.

Also, keep in mind that the risk related to cholesterol increases continuously as the cholesterol level rises. By following the guidelines stringently, one person whose blood cholesterol is 201 may be told that he has a "borderline-high" level, while another person whose result is 199 is told that his cholesterol level is "desirable." Because the readings of these individuals are so close, many doctors will personalize their recommendations, based not solely on the guidelines, but also on each patient's own circumstances (for instance, whether the patient has other risk factors for heart disease, such as smoking or high blood pressure).

The same situation might occur at the higher dividing line. Under the expert panel's guidelines, a person whose cholesterol level is 239 is in the borderline-high zone, while another person with a level of 241 has a high reading. That information may be reassuring to the person with the lower level and extremely frightening for the person with the higher value—when, in reality, their risks regarding cholesterol are almost identical.

The recommendations, then, are simply guidelines. They are not absolutes, and when using them, your doctor will probably make adjustments for factors such as age, sex, heredity and lifestyle.

Again, all other things being equal, the lower your blood cholesterol level, the lower your risk of heart disease. Therefore, any number higher than the one you can *reasonably* achieve with a healthy lifestyle is a number that is too high for you. No matter what cholesterol group you fall into under the guidelines, you should try to get your cholesterol level even lower, as long as it can *reasonably* be done.

Please note the use of the word "reasonably" rather than "possibly." With prescription medications, it is *possible* for almost anyone to reduce his or her blood cholesterol level dramatically—far more than can be achieved with a prudent diet alone. However, the use of drugs usually cannot be justified in a person whose blood cholesterol level is 201, because the potential risks do not justify the potential benefits.

The table turns, however, in someone who cannot get his cholesterol level lower than 250 with diet and exercise alone. In this case, the potential gain with drugs (a 30 to 70 percent reduction in the risk of heart attack or death as the result of coronary heart disease) may well be worth the cost and risks of taking medication.

It becomes even more important to lower your cholesterol level if you have any of the other risk factors for coronary heart disease. Having two or more risk factors at the same time increases the danger enormously. For example, if your cholesterol level is over 240 and you also have high blood pressure, your risk of heart disease may increase six-fold. If, in addition, you smoke, your risk could increase more than twenty times. (The best way to reduce such "combination risks" is to quit smoking and work with your physician to control your blood pressure.)

HDL CHOLESTEROL

How Low Is Too Low?

While lowering your *total* cholesterol is a good idea, it is important to remember that high-density lipoproteins (HDL, or HDL cholesterol) require a different strategy. As you have learned, HDL is one form of cholesterol on which you want to count upward, because it helps to remove cholesterol from the body and can actually prevent the buildup of cholesterol in the walls of your arteries.

Like your total cholesterol, HDL levels are determined in significant part by your heredity. They are also influenced by your age and sex. In children, HDL levels are essentially the same in boys and girls. However, around the time of puberty, HDL levels drop about 20 percent in the boys, and they remain lower in men than in women throughout adult life.

It is more difficult to raise your HDL level than it is to lower your total cholesterol level. Diet can affect HDL levels, but in most studies, dietary changes do not raise HDL levels nearly as much as they lower LDL levels. A high-carbohydrate, low-fat diet will lower LDLs as much as 15 percent but is not likely to raise your HDL levels as much—although there are some exceptions to this general observation. Some researchers have noted that when the total cholesterol level declines markedly, HDL readings decrease as well—an odd and unwelcome paradox for people attempting to improve their cardiovascular health.

No matter what your present risk of coronary heart disease, increasing your HDL level will help lower that risk. High HDL levels can even help you overcome, at least in part, the increased risk of an elevated *total* cholesterol level. In fact, some people with high total cholesterol levels have HDL levels that are also very high—sometimes high enough to completely counterbalance the increased risk of the high total cholesterol. For example, a person who has a total blood cholesterol level of 210 with an HDL of 70 probably has a *lower* risk of heart disease than a person whose total cholesterol level is 200 with an HDL of only 50. The higher you can get your HDL level, the more protection you have against heart disease.

THE EFFECT OF HDL LEVELS ON THE RISK OF CORONARY HEART DISEASE

HDL Level (mg/dl)	Multiplier for Men	Multiplier for Women
30	1.82	—
35	1.49	—
40	1.22	1.94
45	1.00	1.55
50	0.82	1.25
55	0.67	1.00
60	0.55	0.80
65	0.45	0.64
70	—	0.52
75	—	—

The average HDL cholesterol level is 45 for American men and 55 for American women. Since those levels—by definition—will produce an average risk, they are assigned a multiplier value of 1.00. As the HDL level increases, the risk of coronary heart disease drops, and the numerical value of the multiplier goes down. For example, if you are a man and your HDL cholesterol level goes up from 45 to 60, your risk at the new level is only .55 times (55 percent) what it was at the original level. If your HDL level goes down from 45 to 35, your risk of coronary heart disease goes up .49 times (49 percent).

CALCULATING YOUR TOTAL CHOLESTEROL/HDL RATIO

If your doctor follows the National Cholesterol Education Program guidelines, he or she will measure both your total and HDL cholesterol levels as part of a complete lipid profile. With that information in hand, the significance of your HDL level can be estimated—particularly the role it plays in your risk of heart disease—by calculating the ratio between your total cholesterol level and your HDL cholesterol level (the total cholesterol/HDL, or TC/HDL, ratio). For example:

$$\text{If your total cholesterol} = 200 \text{ mg/dl}$$
$$\text{and your HDL cholesterol} = 50 \text{ mg/dl}$$
$$\text{your TC/HDL ratio} = \frac{200}{50} = 4.0$$

The TC/HDL ratio shows you in a mathematical way approximately how much more LDL than HDL is present in your blood. (Remember, in an average person, about 60 to 70 percent of the total cholesterol in the blood is in the form of LDLs.) The more LDL you have in relation to the HDL present, the higher your ratio will be and the higher your risk will be. The less LDL in relation to the HDL present, the lower your ratio and risk will be. These can be clarified by the following two examples:

If your total cholesterol went up and your HDL stayed the same, your total cholesterol/HDL ratio would be higher and your risk of coronary heart disease would be higher than in the example above:

$$\text{If your total cholesterol} = 250 \text{ mg/dl}$$
$$\text{and your HDL cholesterol} = 50 \text{ mg/dl}$$
$$\text{your TC/HDL ratio} = \frac{250}{50} = 5.0$$

If your HDL went up and your total cholesterol stayed the same, your total cholesterol/HDL ratio and your risk of coronary heart disease would be significantly lower than in the initial example:

$$\text{If your total cholesterol} = 200 \text{ mg/dl}$$
$$\text{and your HDL cholesterol} = 60 \text{ mg/dl}$$
$$\text{your TC/HDL ratio} = \frac{200}{60} = 3.33$$

HOW LOW IS LOW ENOUGH FOR THE TC/HDL RATIO?

The average American male has a total cholesterol/HDL ratio of 4.5. In American women, the average ratio is 4.0. (This accounts, at least in part, for the fact that American females have a lower rate of heart disease than males.) But average isn't good enough—the healthiest possible ratio you can *reasonably* achieve is the one you should be seeking.

You can improve (lower) your TC/HDL ratio two ways:

1. Lower your LDL cholesterol level.
2. Raise your HDL level.

You really should try to do both. Changing either one in the right direction will improve your TC/HDL ratio, and changing both will produce dramatic results. As we point out—not only earlier in this section but also in Days 1, 2 and 15—there are many strategies you can use to improve your cholesterol scores. And when you do, your overall vitality will improve, too.

DAY **11** ASSIGNMENTS

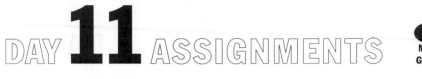

MET GOAL **PARTIALLY MET GOAL** **MISSED GOAL**

PHYSICAL VITALITY

- ○ 1. Improve your time for the measured mile by 2 seconds.   **Time:**_____
- ○ 2. Do all the flexibility and stretching exercises.
- ○ 3. Do the chest, back and arm strength training exercises.

NUTRITIONAL VITALITY

- ○ 4. Decrease total fat intake to 10% of total calories.
- ○ 5. Eat at least 7 half-cup portions of fruits and vegetables.
- ○ 6. Supplement as necessary to reach the vitamin & mineral recommendations.
- ○ 7. Limit dietary cholesterol to 300 mg per day.
- ○ 8. Limit sodium intake to 2,400 mg per day.

MENTAL VITALITY

- ○ 9. Spend at least 10 minutes practicing any deep relaxation technique.
- ○ 10. Identify and eliminate as many sources of stress in your life as you can.

EMOTIONAL & SPIRITUAL VITALITY

MEDICAL VITALITY

SALT   DAY 11

All of us need salt—or more accurately, sodium—to survive. Salt is composed of 40 percent sodium (the other 60 percent is chloride), and our bodies require sodium to properly regulate fluid balance and maintain healthy muscle function.

But when it comes to salt, you can actually get too much of a good thing. Even though sodium is necessary, we certainly don't need very much of it— in fact, less than 500 milligrams of sodium per day. That's only a fraction of a teaspoon of salt.

The National High Blood Pressure Education Program advises healthy individuals to keep their sodium intake below 2,400 milligrams per day. Yet most people consume a lot more than that—about 4,000 milligrams for the average adult. And that excess can sabotage our health. Most notably, it is a major contributor to the development or worsening of high blood pressure in some people.

HYPERTENSION AND SODIUM INTAKE

About 50 million Americans have high blood pressure, or hypertension, although many of them don't know it. In fact, it's often called a "silent disease" because it may cause no symptoms for decades. Your blood pressure reading is a reflection of the force that your circulating blood exerts on the arterial walls. A measurement of 110/70, for example, means that your blood exerts an arterial pressure of 110 mm Hg (millimeters of mercury) as your heart beats (the systolic pressure), and an arterial pressure of 70 mm Hg between heartbeats (diastolic pressure).

To be specific, a reading of 140/90 mm Hg or greater is worrisome, indicating that the pressure of the blood upon your vessel walls is too high. It's not unlike the way that water exerts excessive pressure on the interior walls of a hose when you shut off the nozzle. And if the blood pressure remains high, month after month, year after year, hypertension can scar and damage the inside walls of the arteries and increase the chances of heart disease and stroke. If you also have a high cholesterol level, or if you smoke, the added burden of high blood pressure can further raise your likelihood of a heart attack. At the same time, hypertension forces the heart to work harder, raising the risk of heart failure.

Recent research suggests that your blood pressure goal should be lower than previously recommended. A report from the Framingham Heart Study, published in the *New England Journal of Medicine* in November 2001, indicated that even "high-normal" blood pressure readings significantly increase an individual's risk of a heart attack, stroke, and heart failure. About 13 percent of Americans have these "high-normal" levels, which are a systolic pressure between 130 and 139 mm Hg and/or a diastolic pressure between

85 and 89 mm Hg. The study showed that both men and women with high-normal blood pressure have a 1.5 to 2.5 times greater risk of cardiovascular disease than people with optimal blood pressure readings (120/80 mm Hg or lower).

How does sodium fit into this picture? If you're lucky, sodium has no effect on your blood pressure; in most people, in fact, the kidneys get rid of any extra sodium through the urine. These individuals are called "salt resistant," and their blood pressure remains at healthy levels, no matter how much sodium they consume. But for others, the kidneys do a poor job of eliminating excess sodium; when that happens, the sodium lingering in the blood draws in fluid from the tissues, which increases the volume of fluid in the vessels. That puts extra pressure on the walls of the arteries, driving blood pressure readings upward. As much as 30 percent of the population at large, including about half of those with hypertension, react this way. If you fall into this category, you're "salt-sensitive."

THE BENEFITS OF A LOW-SODIUM DIET

There is plenty of research indicating that by lowering your salt and sodium intake, you may reduce a number of health risks, including your susceptibility to high blood pressure. In 1996, research published in the *British Medical Journal* analyzed data from the massive Intersalt study, which included information on 10,000 people from 32 nations. It concluded that the link between sodium consumption and blood pressure was more powerful than initially believed, especially in middle-aged and elderly populations.

At about the same time, in the *Journal of the American Medical Association*, Canadian researchers published collective data from 56 separate studies. They determined that while sodium does not have a significant influence on people with normal blood pressure readings, a low-sodium diet causes an average four-point decline in systolic blood pressure in people with hypertension. In a separate study involving 2382 men and women at nine major medical centers, researchers documented that by reducing sodium intake, alone or in combination with weight loss, hypertension can be prevented in many men and women. Participants in the study underwent counseling designed to help them lower their sodium intake to 1.8 grams per day and/or reduce their weight. After four years, the incidence of hypertension among these volunteers was about 20 percent lower than a group not undergoing the counseling.

Even modest sodium-related decreases in blood pressure are worth the effort. Remember, the higher your blood pressure, the greater your risk of a heart attack or stroke. A rise in blood pressure of even a few points increases your risk of a heart attack.

In addition to a salt-restricted diet's positive effects on blood pressure, there are other benefits in cutting salt intake. By limiting salt, you can reduce your chances of developing osteoporosis (a weakening of the bones most common in postmenopausal women); that's because excess sodium causes more *calcium* to be excreted in the urine, thus leaving the bones more vulnerable. A study at the University of California at San Francisco reported in 2001 that a high-salt diet (about 4,000 milligrams of sodium per day for four weeks) increased the excretion of urinary calcium by 42 milligrams per day, compared with a low-salt diet (up to 1,500 milligrams of sodium per day)—thus creating a potential calcium deficiency and an increased risk of osteoporosis. Too much sodium can also contribute to kidney stones, and perhaps even to some forms of cancer—most notably, stomach cancer; in countries where salt intake is extremely high, especially where foods are preserved with salt, stomach cancer is much more prevalent than elsewhere in the world.

GETTING SODIUM UNDER CONTROL

It is time to drain the excess sodium from your diet. True, there are a variety of other lifestyle strategies that can also help contribute to *real* vitality, including maintaining a normal weight, exercising regularly, quitting smoking, controlling stress, and maintaining your alcohol intake at moderate levels. But minimizing sodium consumption is also very important. As we've already pointed out, some people are "salt-sensitive," and are more likely to experience increases in blood pressure when excess sodium is consumed. But there are no advantages to a diet soaked in sodium for anyone.

Here is some advice on how to keep your sodium at safe levels:

- Limit the amount of salt you add to your food. Keep the salt shaker off your dining room table, and out of the kitchen while you're cooking.

- When cooking at home, choose fresh, unprocessed foods whenever possible. Emphasize vegetables, fruits, grains and beans in your diet, and you'll fall far below the 2,400-milligram limit of daily sodium. To take the place of salt, season your foods with lemon juice, vinegar, or any number of herbs and spices. Some people find that the pungent taste of pepper reduces any need they once felt for salt. It is remarkable how quickly people get used to food without salt. After a month or two of this way of preparing food, people say that they are actually tasting the real flavor of foods, and have a new appreciation of these natural tastes.

- Try to eat fewer highly-salted snack foods, such as potato chips, corn chips, pretzels and salted nuts; also limit your intake of pickles, olives and soy sauce.

- Cut back on the amount of other processed foods you eat. Even foods that are naturally low in sodium can become high-sodium during manufacturing or canning. These foods include many lunch meats (such as ham, smoked turkey), salad dressings, ketchup, salsa, processed cheeses, canned foods (especially soups), frozen dinners, and gravies. (See the table on the next page for the surprising amount of sodium in foods that may already be in your cupboard and refrigerator.)

SODIUM SURPRISES

While fresh, unprocessed foods are the best choices when you're cutting down on sodium, other foods need to be selected carefully. Scan the list below; you may be surprised at the high levels of sodium found in these common food items.

Baby Food:	**Serving Size**	**Sodium**
Vegetable stew with beef (Gerber Graduates)	6.0 oz	500 mg
Cinnamon animal crackers (Gerber)	3.5 oz	369 mg
Canned Soup:		
Beef with noodles (Progresso)	9.5 oz	1,030 mg
Chicken broth (College Inn)	1 cup	1,320 mg
Clam chowder, New England style (Campbell's), prepared with whole milk	1 cup	930 mg
Tomato (Campbell's), prepared with whole milk	1 cup	740 mg
Condiments:		
BBQ sauce, Hickory Smoke (Kraft)	2 tbsp	440 mg
Catsup (Heinz)	1 tbsp	213 mg
Mustard, Dijon (Grey Poupon)	1 tbsp	450 mg
Mustard, yellow (French's)	1 tbsp	180 mg
Salad Dressing, Italian (Hollywood)	1 tbsp	300 mg
Salad Dressing, Ranch (T. Marzetti), fat-free	1 tbsp	220 mg
Soy sauce (Kikkoman)	1 tbsp	892 mg
Pickles, dill (Vlasic)	1 oz	415 mg
Olives, green, large, with pits, pickled	10 olives	926 mg
Dairy:		
Cheese, grated (Polly-O)	1 oz	530 mg
Cheese, Edam (Kraft)	1 oz	310 mg
Cottage Cheese, creamed, small curd, not packed	1 cup	850 mg
Cottage Cheese, low-fat, 1%, not packed	1 cup	918 mg
Milkshake mix, strawberry (Alba '77 FitN'Prepared)	6 oz	805 mg
Miscellaneous:		
Bagel, plain (Sara Lee)	3.1 oz/1 bagel	580 mg
Baking soda (Arm & Hammer)	1 tsp	952 mg
Biscuit mix (Bisquick)	1/2 cup	700 mg
Rice mix, chicken flavor (Rice-A-Roni)	1/2 cup	560 mg
Pudding, chocolate, instant (Jell-O)	1/2 cup	480 mg

- Look for low-sodium or sodium-free versions of some of your favorite foods. Read the labels on everything you buy. You'll be surprised how many products are now available with very little sodium. Years ago, many people considered these low-sodium products to be flat-tasting—but not anymore. Food manufacturers have learned how to compensate for the missing salt, using spices and other flavorings in its place.

- Talk to your doctor about the prescription medications you are taking; some may contain sodium. Also read the ingredients of over-the-counter medications, which could have sodium in them.

By the way, when you're eating in restaurants, tell the waiter you want your food prepared without added salt, and without sodium-rich condiments and sauces. When choosing salad dressings, a little oil and vinegar is one of your healthiest choices.

DAY **12** ASSIGNMENTS

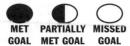

MET GOAL PARTIALLY MET GOAL MISSED GOAL

PHYSICAL VITALITY

○ 1. Improve your time for the measured mile by 2 seconds.   **Time:**_____
○ 2. Do all the flexibility and stretching exercises.
○ 3. Do the leg and abdominal strength training exercises.

NUTRITIONAL VITALITY

○ 4. Decrease total fat intake to 10% of total calories.
○ 5. Eat at least 7 half-cup portions of fruits and vegetables.
○ 6. Supplement as necessary to reach the vitamin & mineral recommendations.
○ 7. Limit dietary cholesterol to 300 mg per day.
○ 8. Limit sodium intake to 2,400 mg per day.

MENTAL VITALITY

○ 9. Spend at least 10 minutes practicing any deep relaxation technique.
○ 10. Identify and eliminate as many sources of stress in your life as you can.

EMOTIONAL & SPIRITUAL VITALITY

○ 11. If you drink alcoholic beverages, limit your daily intake to one drink if you are a woman or 2 drinks if you are a man.

MEDICAL VITALITY

ALCOHOL AND
ALCOHOL ABUSE   DAY 12

About two-thirds of all Americans drink alcoholic beverages. Most are light or moderate drinkers, and for many of them, alcohol can actually have health-promoting benefits. Modest and judicious use of alcohol can improve your cholesterol pattern, reduce your risk of heart attacks, and even decrease your overall chances of mortality.

Early in 1996, the U.S. government's newly issued *Dietary Guidelines for Americans* seemed to give the green light to moderate alcohol intake. For the first time, the guidelines acknowledged that alcohol has possible health benefits, including its ability to protect the cardiovascular system.

Interest in this subject was stimulated greatly by a baffling observation that physicians in France made about their patients. On the one hand, the French consume plenty of saturated fat; even so, their death rate from coronary heart disease is relatively low. This phenomenon, called the "French paradox," led some to suggest that moderate drinking by the French is responsible for their reduced incidence of heart disease.

Could the French affinity for fine wine really explain their reduced mortality due to heart disease? In fact, a number of large studies support the premise that alcohol is heart-friendly; this research shows that a drink or two a day can cut the risk of coronary disease by as much as 20 to 40 percent. In 1995, Harvard investigators reported that moderate alcohol drinkers (just one to three drinks per week) had a 17 percent decreased mortality risk, compared to abstainers. This improvement in longevity was due primarily to fewer deaths from heart attacks. Ironically, heavier drinkers did not fare better. In women who drank a little more—from four drinks per week to about two drinks per day—the reduced risk was 12 percent.

No one is certain how alcohol provides cardioprotection, but a number of factors may play a role. There is consistent evidence, for example, that moderate alcohol intake raises HDL cholesterol—the good cholesterol that can help prevent heart disease—by 10 to 15 percent. There are also data showing that alcohol can help prevent blood clotting, which is a triggering mechanism of heart attacks.

As heartening as this news is, bear in mind that drinking won't do as much for your cardio-fitness as other lifestyle choices discussed in this book, such as regular exercise, cutting your consumption of dietary fat, and reducing your total and LDL ("bad") blood cholesterol levels. And, in addition to the risks of alcoholism discussed throughout this section, there are also other problems associated with drinking. Alcohol increases your risk of developing cancer of the oral cavity, esophagus, and larynx. A 1996 American Cancer Society report cautioned that "cancer risk increases with the amount of alcohol consumed and may start to rise with an intake of as few as two drinks per day." The risk is particularly high in people who both drink and smoke.

For women, perhaps the greatest concern is the link between alcohol and breast cancer—which strikes more than 180,000 women in the United States each year. In some studies, as few as three to nine drinks per week increased the risk of breast cancer by 30 percent; when more than nine drinks were consumed, the risk soared by 60 percent. The cause of this association isn't clear, but it may be related to higher circulating estrogen levels in women who drink.

So how do you achieve a balance between the benefits and the risks of raising a glass of wine at dinner tonight? The American Cancer Society tried to deal with this dilemma in its 1996 guidelines, which suggested that in men over age 50 and in women over age 60, the cardiovascular advantages of alcohol may outweigh the dangers of cancer. However, the report added that "women with an unusually high risk for breast cancer might reasonably consider *abstaining* from alcohol."

About 16 million people drink heavily enough to create serious and potentially life-threatening medical problems, and to warrant the diagnosis of alcoholism. This devastating disease destroys not only individual lives, but also the lives of families. People with this problem are unable to control their drinking, and they develop a physical dependency on alcohol, which is a potent drug. When alcoholics drink, they usually cannot predict when they'll stop, how much they'll drink, or what the consequences of their drinking will be. And, all the while, they often deny the negative effects of drinking upon their lives.

Many of the tragedies that alcohol causes can be avoided by recognizing that a problem exists and making the decision to seek help earlier. The material that follows is designed to help you understand the difference between so-called "social" drinking and problem drinking. The questionnaires in this section will give you an objective way to measure the impact that alcohol is having on your life. They will help you identify whether drinking is creating a problem for you or someone you care about.

THE DIFFERENCES BETWEEN SOCIAL DRINKING AND PROBLEM DRINKING

The drinking patterns of both problem drinkers and moderate, social drinkers can be affected by social and psychological changes in their lives, such as the death of a loved one, the loss of a job, financial difficulties, career pressures, family problems, divorce, loneliness or depression. At some point, however, the drinking patterns of problem drinkers and social drinkers diverge. Social drinkers *occasionally* over-drink and may even become intoxicated. Problem drinkers drink to get drunk on a regular basis. While social drinkers continue to use alcohol as a beverage, problem drinkers begin to use it like a prescription drug, drinking primarily for the medicinal effects. They drink because they want to become intoxicated. They drink to "treat" a hangover. Before long, problem drinkers drink because they cannot stop drinking.

Most social drinkers become less inhibited, more talkative, or deeply relaxed after drinking. But radical changes in their personality do not carry over into the next day. If you are a problem drinker, it's different. Your personality can change dramatically, and other people notice it. You are a gentle person one moment, violent the next. People begin to describe you as "Dr. Jekyll and Mr. Hyde."

There is also a difference in the *amount* of alcohol that social and problem drinkers drink, though that difference is not easily measured. Some social drinkers drink regularly and often and yet never have a problem with alcohol, while some problem drinkers might *appear* to drink quite moderately.

After a while, if you are a problem drinker, you begin to exhibit a deeper and deeper attachment to alcohol. You start planning your life around drinking. You are unhappy in situations where you are unable to drink. You become aware that your drinking is different from most of the people around you. You have to cover up your style of drinking and your method of drinking. You ask yourself, "How can I get at it? How can I get it down? And how can I get rid of the evidence?" You wonder, "How can I get it down faster? How can I keep getting it down without being noticed?" If you are a problem drinker, you have some or all of these warning signs and behavior patterns:

- Need to drink more and more to feel the same effects

- Drink a great deal but do not seem to get drunk

- Do not want to stop drinking

- May stop regularly at a bar after work

- Begin to gulp and sneak drinks

- Switch to harder liquor

- Fail to keep promises to cut down

- May hide liquor in a desk or car

If you are a problem drinker, you increasingly depend on alcohol to get you through problems and to help you forget your troubles. You use alcohol to determine how you will "be" and "feel."

THE PHYSICAL COURSE OF PROBLEM DRINKING

In the earliest stages, problem drinkers develop an increasing tolerance for alcohol. They need more and more alcohol to get the same effect, because their bodies—particularly the nervous system and the liver—learn to adapt to alcohol.

This increased tolerance for alcohol and the body's adaptation to it occur rapidly in some people, but may take years in others, which is why most problem drinkers are able to drink more and more without apparently getting drunk. Anyone who shows an increasing tolerance for alcohol without exhibiting the traditional effects of the drug is on the way to becoming a problem drinker.

In problem drinkers, the body's cells begin to use alcohol for energy. But soon, cells that function well when the blood alcohol level is high are unable to function when the alcohol level drops, and the drinkers' performance deteriorates when their consumption of alcohol goes down. That is when the body has become addicted to alcohol.

In time, the cells and organs that had welcomed alcohol are destroyed by it, and the pleasure of drinking turns into a need to use alcohol as medicine. Once that stage is reached, the problem drinker is sickest when *not* drinking. Physical symptoms of alcohol dependency can include:

- Feeling shaky and agitated, with a gripping desire to remedy this feeling with a drink
- Failure to abstain from alcohol comfortably
- Drinking heavily but rarely getting drunk
- Weakness
- Insomnia
- Vivid dreaming
- Nausea and vomiting
- Fierce hangovers
- Excessive perspiration
- Loss of appetite
- Impairment of memory
- Gagging
- Agitation
- Irritability
- Fast or irregular heartbeat
- Fierce or gross tremors (the shakes)

At this point, the only relief is to drink again—or to call for help. By now, problem drinkers know they ought to stop drinking. In fact, they probably have tried many times. But when they do, they are overwhelmed by painful and frightening withdrawal symptoms—hallucinations, blackouts, DTs (delirium tremens), even convulsions. So they drink again.

Soon, however, even alcohol doesn't work anymore. It may provide relief for a moment or two, but the body loses its tolerance for the drug. Once that happens, only a few drinks can make problem drinkers drunk and sick. Even at this late stage, they can be helped and their bodies can be healed. They can recover. It is never too late, but the longer the drinking goes on, the more difficult it becomes.

THE SOCIAL AND PSYCHOLOGICAL COURSE OF PROBLEM DRINKING

There are some early social and psychological signs that a problem drinker develops. If they are recognized quickly and appropriate action is taken promptly, much of the tragedy that alcohol causes can be avoided. You should be concerned that you are a problem drinker if you:

- Seize any occasion to drink
- Would rather go out drinking than stay home
- Make new friends with heavy drinkers
- Drink to relieve boredom, depression or anxiety, or to otherwise change feelings
- Believe you are drinking in response to serious life stresses
- Feel more charming and sexy when drinking
- Refuse to admit that you have a drinking problem, even though— deep down—you are concerned that you may
- Hide how much you are drinking from others
- Never allow yourself to be caught without a supply of alcohol

Gradually, a problem drinker's involvement with alcohol gets deeper and deeper, and its impact on social life and psychological well-being becomes greater. Even though the problem drinker may still be able to hold a job and support a family financially, the quality of life is rapidly declining. If you are a problem drinker at this stage you:

- Avoid talking about your drinking or become extremely defensive about it
- Become obsessed with drinking as the only way to solve problems and feel good
- Become secretive and deny you are drinking too much
- Use alcohol at odd times of the day and frequently alone
- Become irritable, moody and depressed when not drinking
- Begin to isolate yourself from friends
- Blame your drinking on others
- May become paranoid or resentful of others
- Begin to have marital and family problems
- Spend less and less time with your children
- Lose your sense of self-worth
- Find friends and family making excuses for you
- Feel shame, guilt and remorse for your behavior
- Keep a bottle in your office for spontaneous celebrations
- Begin to have problems at work

Eventually, the traits of a problem drinker become even more conspicuous. As it becomes apparent that you cannot stop drinking, it becomes critically important to you to prove that you can. If you are a problem drinker at this stage you may:

- Switch to beer and wine only (family members who might otherwise pressure you into getting help are often lulled by such tricks)

- Have drastic personality changes and mood swings

- Become disgusted with yourself

- Become irrational, scream, may become violent

- Miss work

- Change jobs or move to a different town

- Drink in the morning, at lunch, and in the middle of the night

- Drink in the car, in the bathroom, even in the closet

- Have blackouts

- Begin to lose interest in sex and have your performance decline

- Show diminished concern for your personal hygiene

- Drink in spite of medical problems made worse by drinking

There comes a point when the problem drinker loses all control and will do anything to avoid the symptoms of withdrawal. At this time, no price seems too great to pay for a drink. If you are a problem drinker at this stage, you:

- Drink just to feel "normal"

- Stop eating regularly

- Go on binges resulting in arrests, hospitalization, and suicide attempts

- Resort to drinking anything that contains alcohol, including cough syrup, rubbing alcohol and shaving lotion

- Avoid everyone you know

- Are wracked by uncontrollable and severe physical withdrawal symptoms

The farther along you progress in this very late stage, the more risk there is of developing permanent physical damage to organs such as your brain and liver. But even at this stage, it is possible to recover with proper treatment.

HOW TO TELL IF YOU'RE DRINKING TOO MUCH

How much is too much? There is no simple answer to that question, because each of us is unique in the way we respond to alcohol and the effects it has on our life. The issue is also an emotional one for many people, so it is difficult to get an objective answer. The questionnaires that follow will help you determine objectively whether drinking is creating a problem for you or someone you care about.

Why take the tests? Because they may show you a problem that you are incapable of recognizing alone. As smart as you may be, as much as you may think you know about this issue, if you are a problem drinker, you simply may not be able to see it yourself.

But even with these questionnaires, you won't see it unless you are completely honest with every answer. It's obvious that you can "cheat" on the tests that follow. If you do, you are only cheating yourself and the people who care about you.

If there are two or more "Yes" answers on any of the tests, you are having problems with alcohol and you should seek professional help immediately.

TEST 1: WHAT IS YOUR RELATIONSHIP WITH ALCOHOL?

Circle the appropriate answer: Y = Yes N = No

Y　N　Does the thought of alcohol cross your mind almost every day?

Y　N　Do you look forward to the next time you can drink?

Y　N　Do you turn more often to friends who also drink?

Y　N　Are you anxious or angry if you have no alcohol available?

Y　N　Is it upsetting to be quizzed about your use of alcohol?

Y　N　Do you prefer that others not know how much or how often you drink?

Y　N　Do you sometimes hate, sometimes love drinking?

Y　N　Are you irritated at suggestions that alcohol is a problem for you?

Y　N　Are you sure that no harm could come to you from your
　　　　use of alcohol if you are careful?

Y　N　Have you changed the form of alcohol you use (e.g., from vodka to beer)
　　　　from time to time, trying to avoid problems of overdoing it?

Y　N　Do you think you may be an abnormal drinker?

_____　Total number of "Yes" answers

TEST 2: WHY DO YOU USE ALCOHOL?

Circle the appropriate answer: Y = Yes N = No

Y   N   Do you drink because you "have to" (business, etc.)?

Y   N   Do you drink on almost every occasion where alcohol is available?

Y   N   Do you drink because you are bored?

Y   N   Do you drink because you are depressed?

Y   N   Do you drink because you are tense?

Y   N   Do you drink to help you sleep?

Y   N   Do you drink to kill physical pain?

Y   N   Do you feel more witty, charming, sexy when you drink?

Y   N   Do you drink because you are shy with people?

Y   N   Do you drink to escape from worry or troubles?

Y   N   Do you drink to increase your energy?

Y   N   Do you drink because you cannot stop drinking?

Y   N   Do you drink to get drunk?

____   **Total number of "Yes" answers**

TEST 3: HOW DO YOU USE ALCOHOL?

Circle the appropriate answer: Y = Yes N = No

Y   N   Do you drink alone?

Y   N   Do you drink differently than those around you?

Y   N   Have you changed your drinking style (e.g., drinking alone or drinking with heavy drinkers) from time to time so as not to be noticed as different?

Y   N   Have you ever hidden a supply of alcohol?

Y   N   Do you cover up the amount you drink?

Y   N   Do you plan for alcohol to be a part of your day as often as possible?

Y   N   Have you mixed alcohol and drugs for a better effect?

Y   N   Do you usually want more than one drink?

Y   N   Do you have a craving to drink at a pretty definite time each day?

____   **Total number of "Yes" answers**

TEST 4: WHAT HAPPENS TO YOUR BRAIN WHEN YOU DRINK?

Circle the appropriate answer: Y = Yes N = No

Y　N　When you drink, do you lose your balance or coordination?

Y　N　When you drink, do you become giddy, silly, talkative, withdrawn?

Y　N　When you drink, do you become argumentative, irritated, or impatient?

Y　N　When you drink, do you become overbearing, depressed, or defensive?

Y　N　Do you undergo a personality change when you drink?

Y　N　Has your efficiency gone down since you began to drink?

Y　N　Have you ever had a loss of memory as a result of drinking
(a blackout, as opposed to passing out)?

Y　N　Have you been unable to cut down or stop drinking?

Y　N　Do you have trouble stopping after starting?

_____ **Total number of "Yes" answers**

TEST 5: WHAT IS DRINKING DOING TO YOUR LIFE?

Circle the appropriate answer: Y = Yes N = No

Y　N　Have you ever felt remorse after drinking?

Y　N　Have you noticed a loss of zest for life?

Y　N　Do you seem to be more disapproving of others now than before?

Y　N　Do other people and life in general seem to be passing you by?

Y　N　Are you frequently feeling guilt and shame?

Y　N　Are your opinions of others stronger and more negative?

Y　N　Have you had thoughts, plans, attempts of suicide?

Y　N　Do you find yourself constantly thinking about yourself?

Y　N　Is shame eating you up?

Y　N　Is drinking upsetting your home life or affecting your job?

Y　N　Is drinking adversely affecting your reputation?

Y　N　Have you gotten into financial difficulties because of your drinking?

Y　N　Has your physician ever treated you for a medical
problem caused by your drinking?

_____ **Total number of "Yes" answers**

GETTING HELP FOR PROBLEM DRINKERS

We are finally beginning to understand why some people can drink regularly and never have a problem with alcohol, while others end up as problem drinkers. Researchers began to suspect a hereditary factor when they discovered that children of alcoholics were four times more likely to become addicted to alcohol than children whose parents had no trouble with drinking. To be sure that the problem wasn't caused by growing up in a bad environment, they studied children whose natural parents were alcoholic, but who were raised in adoptive homes without alcoholic parents. These children, too, were more likely to become addicted to alcohol, which showed that the tendency toward alcoholism is hereditary.

Further research supports this belief. Studies show that the brain of an alcoholic responds differently to alcohol than the brain of a non-alcoholic, and research with children of alcoholics shows that their brains often react differently. It is this difference in the way the brain reacts to alcohol that enables some people to enjoy a drink without problems, while others are literally drawn into alcohol's addictive web.

Historically, alcoholics were always seen as morally weak—a blight on family and society. Everyone thought that the town drunk had no one to blame for ruining his life but himself, and alcoholic women were viewed with even greater disdain. Even today, many people see alcoholism as a moral or psychological issue—in spite of the scientific evidence for biological susceptibility. They believe that problem drinkers abuse alcohol because they don't manage life's problems like normal people.

There is no doubt that psychological, cultural, and social factors influence an alcoholic's drinking. But it is no longer possible to ignore the underlying genetic and physical foundation for this disease. In this regard, it helps to think of alcoholism as a disorder of the brain, just as allergies are a disorder of the immune system. Recovering problem drinkers must avoid alcohol just as allergic persons must avoid pollens.

Given the damage that problem drinking can cause if left untreated, you would expect every problem drinker to rush for help. Unfortunately, help is almost never sought. Rarely do problem drinkers accept the notion that something that makes them feel so good, that seems to solve so many problems, that is so much a part of daily life, can also eventually destroy them. Besides, most alcoholics are still functional, earning a living, and supporting their families—at least financially. The false appearance of normalcy makes it easier for them to say to themselves and to others that they do not really have a problem with alcohol.

Family and friends delude themselves, too, denying the seriousness of the situation and hoping for some kind of spontaneous change to happen. It rarely does. And through their denial and inaction, they actually allow the problem to continue. There is something about alcohol that destroys everyone's ability to make sensible decisions, or to even see that a problem exists. Alcohol enables alcoholics to deny reality, and it paralyzes the people around them from doing anything about it. So most alcoholics "bottom out" before anything is done. They lose their jobs and their families, and destroy their health and self-respect before they admit there is a problem and take the steps that will lead to recovery. Some never live to take those steps.

Almost anyone, from a spouse or a child to a friend or employer, can initiate an alcoholic's recovery program. It can be difficult, though. Typically, each of these people has been drawn into the web of denial and deception that allowed the alcoholic to reach this point. It is time now for everyone to adopt new behaviors.

One of the most effective techniques for motivating a problem drinker to start treatment is an organized "intervention," in which all of the important individuals in the person's life come together to confront the issue and offer love and support. Taking this kind of unified stand is often the only way to make someone with an alcohol-affected brain understand the seriousness of the problem and decide to go into treatment. An intervention is usually best done with the guidance of a professional intervention counselor.

The problem drinker is physically and emotionally sick. As difficult as it may be, family and friends must refuse to participate any longer in the sick pattern of fear, guilt, shame, anger and pity that inevitably accompanies this illness.

Where To Go For Treatment

The primary treatment resources include comprehensive treatment programs (both inpatient and outpatient) and Alcoholics Anonymous (AA) groups. There are treatment programs everywhere, and there are AA groups in almost every community.

Treatment Programs

Experience has shown that the best and most successful treatment programs include:

- A period of detoxification

- A minimum of four weeks of patient care, either inpatient or outpatient

- Intensive nutritional therapy and education

- Strong emphasis on AA participation for long-term sobriety

- Thorough follow-up care

- Involvement of the family in treatment and follow-up

Some people can recover by going to Alcoholics Anonymous alone, but medical supervision and detoxification are often necessary to start a person on the road to recovery. For this reason, many people find it necessary to participate in a comprehensive, structured treatment program. Most of these programs are covered by health insurance or government-supported medical aid programs.

If a person's commitment to recovery is exceptionally strong, and the environment at home is extremely supportive, it is possible to undergo treatment as an outpatient, sleeping at home at night. When these conditions are not met, it is advisable that an inpatient program be used. A physician or alcoholism counselor can be very helpful in deciding which approach is more appropriate for a particular person.

Nutrition is an important part of any treatment program, since most problem drinkers are chronically malnourished. In addition to a well-balanced diet, vitamin and mineral supplements are usually needed to help correct the years of physical damage that long-term alcohol abuse has wrought on the body.

Alcoholics Anonymous (AA)

Alcoholics Anonymous describes itself as "a fellowship of men and women who share their experience, strength and hope with each other that they may solve their common problem and help others to recover from alcoholism. ... Our primary purpose is to stay sober and help other alcoholics achieve sobriety." The only requirement for membership is a desire to stop drinking. There are no dues or fees for AA membership. AA is not allied with any sect, denomination, political group, organization or institution.

All AA members share the disease of alcoholism and are committed to helping themselves and each other to live happy, constructive, alcohol-free lives. Through the support, camaraderie, and experiences shared at AA meetings, members are able to express and release the feelings, problems and fears that formerly accompanied their drinking.

Members of AA must admit their powerlessness over alcohol. AA is not a religious organization, nor does it require a traditional belief in God. It does, however, require a willingness to accept the notion of a "higher power." Some people in AA use God as their higher power, some use the mysteries of the universe and nature. Others find that believing in the power of a group of people serves their purpose and helps them to stay sober.

In AA, members find constant support and help from others who understand and share the very same problem. AA members frequently ask another, more experienced member to "sponsor" them—to guide them through the Twelve Steps of the AA program and help them develop their own personal path to recovery. Working through the Twelve Steps of Alcoholics Anonymous helps bring about the changes necessary to deal with the problems of living without alcohol.

AA is a lifelong program. Alcoholics are never considered "cured." With the help and support of AA, they practice *recovery* for the rest of their lives.

If you think you have a problem with alcohol, one of the best things you can do is visit an AA meeting and ask for help. You can find the times and locations of meetings by calling the nearest AA central office. Every telephone book has a listing for Alcoholics Anonymous in the white or yellow pages. You can also get the number by calling the local telephone information operator.

Al-Anon

Al-Anon is a program for the family members and friends of a problem drinker or of a practicing or recovering alcoholic. Like AA, Al-Anon works through group support. Members attend meetings and share their feelings and experiences with others who have lived through similar situations. Al-Anon members learn that alcoholism is a family disease that affects everyone around the alcoholic. Al-Anon helps family members and friends break out of the destructive patterns and dependencies that they have become accustomed to and enables them to live happy and productive lives.

Al-Anon teaches family members and friends how to help the problem drinker in an appropriate manner. It also teaches them to focus on their own needs first. Al-Anon members learn that by helping themselves, they are helping the person with an alcohol problem. This lesson is necessary if they are ever to have happy and fulfilling lives, with or without the problem drinker.

Al-Anon members meet together in both small and large groups. They also exchange phone numbers so that support and help are only a phone call away. Like AA members, new Al-Anon members are encouraged to ask another, more experienced member to "sponsor" them—to guide them through the Twelve Steps of the Al-Anon program, and to help them develop their own personal path to recovery.

If you are a family member or friend of a problem drinker in need of help or someone to talk to, you can get information about Al-Anon meetings near you by calling Alcoholics Anonymous or looking up Al-Anon in your phone book. You can also call the Al-Anon headquarters for information about Al-Anon programs in your area (Al-Anon World Service Office: 1-800-344-2666).

A FINAL NOTE

Problem drinkers are ordinary people whose bodies and brains are unable to handle alcohol in an ordinary way. They cannot be blamed for their genetic susceptibility to alcohol. But they must shoulder the responsibility for the consequences if they do nothing about their problem.

It is difficult to admit that a drinking problem exists, and harder still to correct it. But taking the necessary steps to recovery is well worth the trouble and pain. It is the only way to regain your happiness and self-respect.

If you or someone you care about has a problem with alcohol, make the commitment to start the recovery process now. It is never too late—or too early—to take the first step.

DAY 13 ASSIGNMENTS

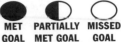

MET GOAL   **PARTIALLY MET GOAL**   **MISSED GOAL**

PHYSICAL VITALITY

○ 1. Improve your time for the measured mile by 2 seconds.   **Time:_____**

○ 2. Do all the flexibility and stretching exercises.

NUTRITIONAL VITALITY

○ 3. Decrease total fat intake to 10% of total calories.

○ 4. Eat at least 7 half-cup portions of fruits and vegetables.

○ 5. Supplement as necessary to reach the vitamin & mineral recommendations.

○ 6. Limit dietary cholesterol to 300 mg per day.

○ 7. Limit sodium intake to 2,400 mg per day.

MENTAL VITALITY

○ 8. Spend at least 10 minutes practicing any deep relaxation technique.

○ 9. Identify and eliminate as many sources of stress in your life as you can.

EMOTIONAL & SPIRITUAL VITALITY

○ 10. If you drink alcoholic beverages, limit your daily intake to one drink if you are a woman or 2 drinks if you are a man.

MEDICAL VITALITY

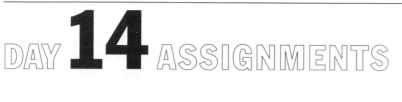

DAY **14** ASSIGNMENTS

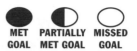

MET GOAL **PARTIALLY MET GOAL** **MISSED GOAL**

PHYSICAL VITALITY

○ 1. Improve your time for the measured mile by 2 seconds.   **Time**:_____

○ 2. Do all the flexibility and stretching exercises.

○ 3. Do the chest, back and arm strength training exercises.

NUTRITIONAL VITALITY

○ 4. Decrease total fat intake to 10% of total calories.

○ 5. Eat at least 7 half-cup portions of fruits and vegetables.

○ 6. Supplement as necessary to reach the vitamin & mineral recommendations.

○ 7. Limit dietary cholesterol to 300 mg per day.

○ 8. Limit sodium intake to 2,400 mg per day.

MENTAL VITALITY

○ 9. Spend at least 10 minutes practicing any deep relaxation technique.

○ 10. Identify and eliminate as many sources of stress in your life as you can.

EMOTIONAL & SPIRITUAL VITALITY

○ 11. If you drink alcoholic beverages, limit your daily intake to one drink if you are a woman or 2 drinks if you are a man.

MEDICAL VITALITY

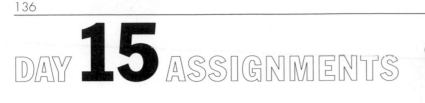

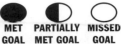

PHYSICAL VITALITY

○ 1. Improve your time for the measured mile by 2 seconds.   **Time:_____**

○ 2. Do all the flexibility and stretching exercises.

○ 3. Do the leg and abdominal strength training exercises.

NUTRITIONAL VITALITY

○ 4. Decrease total fat intake to 10% of total calories.

○ 5. Eat at least 7 half-cup portions of fruits and vegetables.

○ 6. Supplement as necessary to reach the vitamin & mineral recommendations.

○ 7. Limit dietary cholesterol to 300 mg per day.

○ 8. Limit sodium intake to 2,400 mg per day.

○ 9. Consume at least 25 grams of dietary fiber per day.

MENTAL VITALITY

○ 10. Spend at least 10 minutes practicing any deep relaxation technique.

○ 11. Identify and eliminate as many sources of stress in your life as you can.

EMOTIONAL & SPIRITUAL VITALITY

○ 12. If you drink alcoholic beverages, limit your daily intake to one drink if you are a woman or 2 drinks if you are a man.

MEDICAL VITALITY

FIBER   DAY 15

"Eat your fruits and vegetables!"

You—and many millions of other people—were probably raised on that motherly advice. But now, there is finally plenty of science to support it. In fact, mother was right: The fiber in fruits and vegetables—and in many other healthy foods—is a powerful tool for preventing disease and improving your overall fitness level. Research around the world shows that consuming fiber decreases your risk of heart disease, colon cancer, diabetes, and constipation. And if you're trying to lose weight, fiber can help; not only are fiber-rich foods low in fat, but they are filling (even though they're relatively low in calories). They also tend to require more chewing, so they make you eat more slowly.

WHAT IS FIBER?

Fiber is a substance found only in plant foods. This part of the plant is resistant to the body's digestive tract enzymes; as a result, only a relatively small amount of fiber is digested or metabolized in the stomach or intestines, and thus most of it passes through the stomach and small intestine intact.

There are two main types of fiber—soluble and insoluble—categorized by whether they dissolve in water. Most foods contain a mixture of both. Although fiber provides the body with no nutrients in its own right, it still is an important component of our diets. Researchers credit soluble fiber with lowering cholesterol and the risk of heart disease. On the other hand, the insoluble variety provides protection against some forms of cancer; it absorbs many times its weight in water, so stools (and their toxic substances) pass through the intestines more easily and rapidly.

Here are just some of the specific ways that fiber contributes to physical fitness:

- **Heart Disease.** Fiber-rich foods are naturally low in dietary fat and cholesterol. That in itself will help lower your blood cholesterol levels. But fiber also seems to have the power to accelerate the elimination of bile acids (cholesterol breakdown products) through the stool, thus strengthening the anti-cholesterol knockout punch.

    One of the most persuasive recent studies on fiber came out of Harvard University, where scientists have been studying the health of more than 51,000 male health professionals. In data published in 1996, researchers evaluated the heart-attack risk of men consuming various levels of dietary fiber. Their conclusion: Among men in the top fifth of fiber consumption, their chances of having a heart attack were 36 percent lower than those in the bottom fifth. The greatest protection came from fiber found in grains such as cold breakfast cereal—a 27 percent reduced risk for a 10-gram daily increase in cereal fiber; those men who ate at least seven servings of fruits and vegetables a day had a 22 percent lower likelihood of experiencing a heart attack.

- **Constipation.** By adding bulk to stools, fiber helps produce softer stools that move easily through the digestive tract, preventing constipation.

- **Colon Cancer.** As softer stools are transported more rapidly through the digestive system, the colon has less exposure to fecal carcinogens (cancer-causing substances). Fiber also soaks up bile acids, which appear to play a role in the development of cancer when they are present at high levels. A large study published in the *Journal of the National Cancer Institute* in 1992 concluded that a high-fiber, low-fat diet can help prevent the growth of precancerous polyps in the colon lining.

- **Diabetes.** When it comes to diabetes and fiber, there is good news. A high-fiber diet helps reduce blood-sugar levels in people who already have the disease. Studies also show that population groups without diabetes who eat plenty of fiber tend to have a lower risk of developing the disease, compared to population groups without diabetes who consume smaller amounts of fiber. Researchers believe that soluble fiber may slow the rate at which sugar is absorbed from the small intestine.

HOW MUCH DO YOU NEED?

The National Research Council recommends an intake of at least 25 to 35 grams of dietary fiber each day, while the National Cancer Institute calls for 25 to 30 grams. Nevertheless, most Americans are eating a fiber-deficient diet, even though plenty of tasty, attractive and inexpensive high-fiber foods are widely available. The average adult now consumes only about 12 grams of dietary fiber a day—not nearly enough to have a positive effect on your high cholesterol level, for example.

What's the easiest and best way to get the fiber you need? Simply eat a variety of foods—brown rice, fruits, vegetables, oat bran, breads, and beans and other legumes. Five servings of fruits and vegetables will give you an average of about 17 grams a day, which is a good head start toward your fiber goal. Also begin reading labels, which will tell you the amount of total fiber in a serving of packaged food.

Here are some other tips for filling up on fiber:

- Several times a week, rather than eating animal products, substitute food from plants instead. For example, eat beans instead of beef.

- Rather than drinking fruit juice, eat the whole fresh fruit (which contains much more fiber). Choose whole-grain alternatives instead of refined grain products (processing decreases the fiber content). For example, select brown rice rather than white rice.

- Eat the skin and the membranes of fruits and vegetables (such as apples, pears, potatoes, tomatoes, and carrots), and consume the stems of vegetables like broccoli.

- Use corn tortillas rather than white flour tortillas.

- Enjoy some air-popped popcorn or a dish of fresh fruit as a late-night snack.

- If you experience unwelcome bloating and intestinal gas when you add fiber to the diet, you can minimize this embarrassing problem by increasing your intake gradually, adding one to two grams a day.

FIBER SOURCES

Food	Approximate Grams of Fiber
Apple–raw, unpeeled, 1 medium or Apricot–raw, halves, 1 cup	3.7
Boysenberry–unsweetened, 1 cup	5.2
Raspberry–trimmed, 1 cup	8.4
Strawberry–trimmed, 1 cup	3.9
Orange–Florida, 1 medium	3.6
Pear–untrimmed, 1 medium	10.9
Prunes–dried, 1 cup	11.6
Cabbage–raw, 1/12 head, or Cauliflower–fresh, 1/6 head	2.0
Carrot 1 medium	2.3
Broccoli–boiled, drained, 4 oz.	2.9
Black Beans–boiled, 1/2 cup	7.5
Black-Eyed Peas–boiled, drained	10.9
Kidney Beans or Pinto Beans–canned, 1/2 cup	5.0
Navy Beans–canned, 1/2 cup	7.0
Spinach–raw, 3 oz.	8.0
Corn–cooked, 1/2 cup	3.4
Brussels Sprouts–boiled, drained, 4 oz.	4.9
Barley–pearled, cooked, 4 oz.	4.5
Bran–1/3 cup	8.0
Oat Bran–Quaker, 1 oz.	4.2
Wheat Bran, 1 oz.	10.1
Bran Flakes, 1 oz.	5.0
Oats–cooked, 1 cup	3.5
Wheat Bran–toasted, 1 oz.	11.4
Whole-Wheat Bread–100%, 1 slice	2.0
Bran Muffin–with raisins, 1 muffin	4.0

DAY 16 ASSIGNMENTS

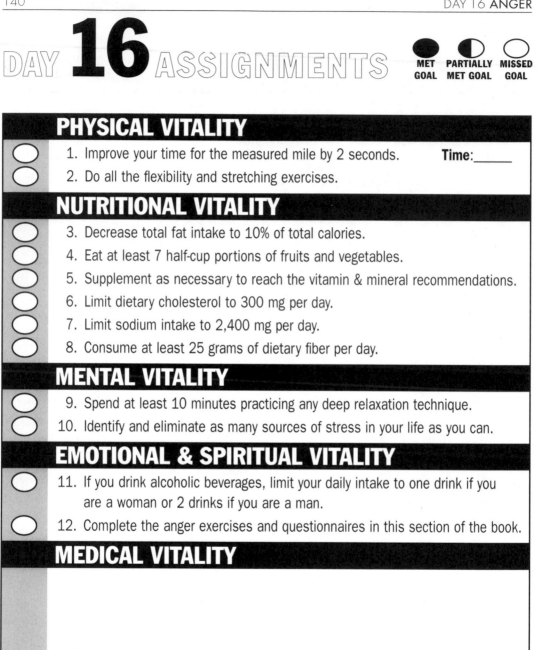

● MET GOAL   ◑ PARTIALLY MET GOAL   ○ MISSED GOAL

PHYSICAL VITALITY

○
○

1. Improve your time for the measured mile by 2 seconds.   **Time:_____**
2. Do all the flexibility and stretching exercises.

NUTRITIONAL VITALITY

3. Decrease total fat intake to 10% of total calories.
4. Eat at least 7 half-cup portions of fruits and vegetables.
5. Supplement as necessary to reach the vitamin & mineral recommendations.
6. Limit dietary cholesterol to 300 mg per day.
7. Limit sodium intake to 2,400 mg per day.
8. Consume at least 25 grams of dietary fiber per day.

MENTAL VITALITY

9. Spend at least 10 minutes practicing any deep relaxation technique.
10. Identify and eliminate as many sources of stress in your life as you can.

EMOTIONAL & SPIRITUAL VITALITY

11. If you drink alcoholic beverages, limit your daily intake to one drink if you are a woman or 2 drinks if you are a man.
12. Complete the anger exercises and questionnaires in this section of the book.

MEDICAL VITALITY

ANGER

DAY 16

This section of our program will teach you things you can do to manage your anger more effectively, but it is not designed to treat serious emotional disorders. If anger is creating serious problems in your life and you are unable to improve the way you feel by using the tools in these pages, you should consult your family doctor or a mental health professional for further help and advice. This information should not be used in place of medical treatment, psychotherapy or counseling when they are indicated.

Anger is an emotion that every human being experiences from infancy onward. It's almost impossible to avoid being angry. But many people try to cover up their anger. They don't like to admit they are angry, because they were taught as children that angry feelings were "bad." But feelings are not "good" or "bad." They are signals that let you and others know in a very truthful way what you are really experiencing. Angry feelings should not be ignored or covered up.

But anger cannot just be let loose either. Like all emotions, it causes both psychological and physical reactions that can have serious negative effects on your health and well-being and on the health and well-being of those around you. Mismanaged anger can adversely affect just about every aspect of your life. It can ruin your physical and mental health, your relationships with loved ones, and your performance at work. For example, a 1996 study reported in *Circulation* concluded that older men with high levels of anger may have triple the risk of heart disease than men with much lower anger levels. Other studies have shown a significant association between anger and hypertension and stroke.

It is not the anger itself that is damaging. It is the mismanagement of anger that can get you in trouble. Mismanaged anger distorts your thinking and disrupts your thoughts and actions. It causes you to act impulsively and aggressively, and to do things you will regret later. It almost always promotes a negative impression on others.

But you don't have to let anger disrupt your life and hurt others. In the following pages, you will learn how to manage anger in a more constructive way. You will find a seven-step program that will help you recognize the early signs of anger and do something about your anger before it gets out of control. You'll learn how to measure the amount of anger in your life, and how to create a plan of action that channels your anger in more productive directions. You will learn more about what triggers your anger, and be introduced to techniques and interventions you can use to control it more effectively. By gaining more control over anger, you'll be taking a giant step toward *real* vitality.

EVALUATING YOUR ANGER

There are four questions you must answer before you can manage your anger effectively: Is your anger valid? Is it needless? Is it just? Is it a problem?

When Anger Is Valid

Anger is *always* valid. Instead of feeling guilty about getting angry, you should accept the fact that you *are* angry and start dealing with the reality of it. The more you learn to accept your anger as something you are entitled to feel, the less trouble it will cause you.

When Anger Is Needless

Needless anger is anger that makes a situation worse. When anger causes you to lash out destructively, when it causes you to get upset about things you cannot avoid or change, it is needless. A simple way to tell if your anger is needless is to ask yourself, "Is my anger helping me in this situation or is it hurting me?" If it's hurting you, your anger is needless in the sense that you need to develop a more productive response to the situation.

Anger is useful when it causes you to take a positive action. It can motivate you to solve an irritating problem. It can signal you that something wrong is happening. It can stimulate you to take charge of a situation.

When Anger Is Just

Anger is just when there is a good reason for it—when it occurs in response to someone who has intentionally and unnecessarily acted in a way that could hurt you (for example, someone who has lied to you or betrayed you). Anger is unjust when it is caused by someone who had no intention of hurting you, or when there is a good reason for the situation that has provoked you (for example, cancellation of a flight due to bad weather), or because you have distorted the situation.

The more unjust your anger is, the more likely you will be to regret it later and the more destructive its effects are likely to be. The more your anger is just, the better you will feel about the times you are angry (although anger itself never feels good). However, even when your anger is just, you cannot express it in an unjust manner and expect to feel good about things afterward. Regardless of the cause for your anger, responding in a hurtful way will only aggravate the situation.

When Anger Is A Problem

Anger is becoming a problem when it occurs too often; when it feels too intense; when it lasts too long; when it makes you act in a destructive way; when it keeps you from doing your work; and when it hurts your relationships with others.

IF YOU WANT FURTHER GUIDANCE...

The seven-step anger management program that follows is based on the scientific work and clinical experience of Dr. Hendrie Weisinger, whose comprehensive approach to anger management has been used successfully for many years by individuals and employers. If, after using the introductory program in this book, you wish to go further with this approach, you should consider reading the books written by Dr. Weisinger. They include: *Dr. Weisinger's Anger Work-Out Book* and *Anger at Work: Learning the Art of Anger Management on the Job.*

SEVEN STEPS FOR MANAGING ANGER

Anger is a complex reaction, involving thoughts and actions as well as feelings. Anger is so complex, it can be difficult to manage unless you break the problem down into smaller, more manageable parts. Here are the seven steps of our *Anger Management Program*:

> *Step 1: Monitoring Your Anger*
> *Step 2: Learning What Makes You Angry*
> *Step 3: Getting Rid of Anticipatory Anger*
> *Step 4: Getting Rid of Past Anger*
> *Step 5: Solving Your Problems*
> *Step 6: Building a Support System*
> *Step 7: Anger Management Interventions*

STEP 1: MONITORING YOUR ANGER

Most people get angry far more often than they realize even people who don't have serious problems with anger. The average person gets angry a dozen times a day. You may say, "No, not me." But what about those seconds of irritation when you try to make a phone call and get a busy signal? What about the irritation you feel while stuck in traffic or standing in line at the supermarket? All those minutes add up and have their negative effects.

In order to really know how anger is affecting your life, you've got to monitor your angry episodes, so you'll know how often you are getting angry each day and how upsetting each episode of anger is to you. You also need to have this information so you can tell if the *Anger Management Program* is working for you.

There is a fascinating side effect that occurs when people begin to monitor their behavior carefully: Without even trying, their behavior begins to change in ways that are usually desirable.

There are two ways to monitor the amount of anger you are experiencing:

- Self-monitoring (accurately observing your own behavior)
- Observation by others (to validate your observations)

Self-Monitoring Anger

There are several things you can measure to learn how anger is affecting your life:

- How often it occurs (the frequency)

- How long it lasts (the duration)

- How intense it feels (the intensity)

- How just it is

- How well you manage it

Just measuring these factors is not enough; you also must keep a written record of your observations. This is the only way you can follow your progress over time and be sure that this *Anger Management Program* is really working for you.

The *Daily Anger Diary* will give you a simple way to keep track of all the things you should be monitoring. Carry the diary with you and make an entry in it every time you feel yourself getting angry, or make notes on scratch paper that you can transfer later to the diary. You will find a blank diary page on page 146. Make enough photocopies of it to last the duration of the program.

Your *Anger Score*, which you will calculate in the diary, is an approximation of the amount of time you spend each day feeling angry. It also takes into account the intensity of your anger. To calculate your *Anger Score*, write down in the diary every incident during the day that creates feelings of anger or irritation. Then quantify the anger by entering the number of minutes each episode lasts and assigning a value to the intensity of your feelings. Next, by multiplying the number of minutes times the intensity value, you'll get the *Anger Score* for that episode. Finally, calculate your *Anger Score* for the day by adding up all of the individual scores.

The diary also provides you with a simple mechanism for monitoring how much of the anger you feel is just or unjust and how well or poorly you managed each episode.

Observation By Others

If you are truly honest with yourself about the anger you are experiencing and you are very diligent about making entries, the *Anger Diaries* will provide you with an accurate measure of your progress with this *Anger Management Program*. However, it's human nature to ignore some episodes of anger, or to forget to record them, so you may want to ask another person to help you by providing independent observations. Obviously, that person won't be able to observe you 24 hours a day, and may not be aware of all the times when you are feeling angry. Still, having someone verify your observations for even a few hours may reveal the need for you to monitor yourself more carefully.

Here is a sample page to show you how to make entries in the *Daily Anger Diary* on page 146. Make enough copies of the Diary page to last at least until the end of your program (12 copies).

SAMPLE DAILY ANGER DIARY PAGE

Time	Cause	Minutes x Intensity = Anger Score			Just or Unjust	Managed Well/Poorly
7am	Normal Traffic (A.M.)	25 x 2	=	50	U	P
9:15	Office Argument	5 x 2	=	10	U	W
12:30	Lunch Argument	15 x 4	=	60	J	P
1:30	Argument with Boss	30 x 4	=	120	U	P
4:55	Traffic Jam (P.M.)	45 x 5	=	225	U	P
7:20	Argument with Kids	5 x 3	=	15	J	W
9:15	Argument with Wife	60 x 4	=	240	U	P
TOTALS:		185		720	2/5	2/5

Anger Intensity Level:
    1 = Minimal anger; fairly relaxed
    2 = Slight anger; showing some temper
    3 = Moderate anger; begins to lose temper
    4 = High anger; temper lost
    5 = Severe anger; loses all control

Date: _____

DAILY ANGER DIARY				
Time	Cause	Minutes x Intensity = Anger Score	Just or Unjust	Managed Well/Poorly
		X =		
		X =		
		X =		
		X =		
		X =		
		X =		
		X =		
		X =		
		X =		
		X =		
		X =		
		X =		
		X =		
		X =		
		X =		
		X =		
		X =		
		X =		
TOTALS:				

Anger Intensity Level: 1 = Minimal anger; fairly relaxed
2 = Slight anger; showing some temper
3 = Moderate anger; begins to lose temper
4 = High anger; temper lost
5 = Severe anger; loses all control

STEP 2: LEARNING WHAT MAKES YOU ANGRY

Each time you make an entry in the *Daily Anger Diary*, you'll write down the particular thing that triggered each episode of anger. After you've done this for a few days, you should have enough entries to let you determine which triggers are repeatedly causing you to become angry. Once you become aware of your anger triggers, you can take steps to avoid them, when possible, and you can learn a different way of reacting to them when they can't be avoided.

Most anger triggers can be put into one of the following categories:

- Frustrations—you are prevented or blocked from doing something you wanted, or you are disappointed by someone or something

- Irritations and annoyances—incidents that get on your nerves, such as noise or frequent interruptions

- Abuse—verbal or physical

- Injustice or unfairness—situations where you believe you have been treated unfairly

Once you have made at least twenty entries into the *Daily Anger Diary*, review the *Cause* column and identify the anger triggers that occur repeatedly. List your five most common triggers below, and describe–as best you can–what it is about each one that makes you angry:

1. _____

   _____

   _____

2. _____

   _____

   _____

3. _____

   _____

   _____

4. _____

   _____

   _____

5. _____

   _____

   _____

STEP 3: GETTING RID OF ANTICIPATORY ANGER

Often, anger arises because of unmet expectations. When these expectations are reasonable (for example, expecting someone to pay a debt on time), the anger is just and it may even produce the desired results next time. When the expectations are unrealistic (for example, expecting a promotion when there isn't a vacancy), the anger that arises will be unjust, needless, and unproductive.

But some people get angry even *before* the disappointment occurs, because they expect to be disappointed. For example, you expect someone who has always been late for appointments to show up late again, so you get angry before the person is due to arrive. Even if that individual shows up on time, it's too late because your anger is already there. Getting angry before anything has really happened—because you expect it to happen—is referred to as anticipatory anger.

This anticipatory anger creates its own vicious cycle of anger, because the other person reacts to your unjust anger by getting angry, too. It's especially destructive when the other individual is attempting to change the behavior that is provoking your anger. Your anticipatory anger will make the other person believe that it's not worth the effort.

The worksheet that follows will help you identify people and situations that are responsible for your feeling anticipatory anger. Use it to determine what expectations are causing your anger and whether those expectations are reasonable and realistic. The worksheet will also help you develop an action plan to stop the vicious cycle of anticipatory anger at its source. Make photocopies of the opposite page to deal with the people and situations that most commonly cause anticipatory anger for you.

SAMPLE ANTICIPATORY ANGER WORKSHEET

Name a person or situation that almost always seems to make you angry.

My mother

What is it that makes you angry?

I just know she's going to criticize me

Is it realistic to expect that person or situation to change? ☐ Yes ☒ No

If yes, how are you going to make that change come about? If no, what changes will you make yourself so you stop getting angry all the time?

1. I'll be honest with her and tell her how bad her criticisms make me feel.

2. I'll do my yoga exercises before she comes to release some of the tension I feel ahead of time.

ANTICIPATORY ANGER WORKSHEET

Name a person or situation that almost always seems to make you angry.

_____

What is it that makes you angry?

_____

Is it realistic to expect that person or situation to change? ☐ *Yes* ☐ *No*

If yes, how are you going to make that change come about? If no, what changes will you make yourself so you stop getting angry all the time?

_____

_____

ANTICIPATORY ANGER WORKSHEET

Name a person or situation that almost always seems to make you angry.

_____

What is it that makes you angry?

_____

Is it realistic to expect that person or situation to change? ☐ *Yes* ☐ *No*

If yes, how are you going to make that change come about? If no, what changes will you make yourself so you stop getting angry all the time?

_____

_____

ANTICIPATORY ANGER WORKSHEET

Name a person or situation that almost always seems to make you angry.

_____

What is it that makes you angry?

_____

Is it realistic to expect that person or situation to change? ☐ *Yes* ☐ *No*

If yes, how are you going to make that change come about? If no, what changes will you make yourself so you stop getting angry all the time?

_____

_____

STEP 4: GETTING RID OF PAST ANGER

You may be plagued by anger that persists long after the incident that caused the anger has passed. Usually this occurs because the original incident was so upsetting that you covered it up and tried to bury the feelings associated with it. But your mind cannot truly hide something that upsetting. Until you deal with this past anger once and for all, it will continue to spoil the quality of your life. The best way to overcome this problem is to let the feelings out—to experience them fully and honestly.

There are six ways you can deal with these feelings:

- Acknowledge them

- Share them

- Act them out

- Document them

- Make peace with the source of your anger

- Let the feelings go

Acknowledging Your Angry Feelings

The hardest part of dealing with past anger is admitting that something that happened so long ago can still be upsetting to you. Most of us like to think we are stronger than that, but none of us is immune from it.

Take time now to list the sources of your past anger. You may find this difficult, because doing so can stir up all of the anger and other feelings you've been hiding. You must do it, though, if you are ever going to eliminate past anger as a source of unhappiness in the future.

The worksheet on the opposite page contains room for recording three sources of past anger and identifying the reasons why you have been unable to overcome it. You can photocopy this worksheet or use loose sheets of paper to write down other sources of past anger.

Sharing Your Angry Feelings

Many people have problems with past angry feelings because they are ashamed of these feelings or embarrassed by them, so they try to hide their feelings from other people. If you allow yourself to do this, you not only magnify the unjustified shame and embarrassment, but you also deprive yourself of an important source of support for what you are feeling.

The best way to deal with past angry feelings is to share them openly and honestly with someone you trust and who cares about you. Do not share your feelings with anyone who criticizes them or your right to feel the way you do. The other person is not there to

PAST ANGER WORKSHEET

I am still angry about _____

_____

_____

I have been unable to overcome this anger because it makes me feel:

_____

_____

_____

I am still angry about _____

_____

_____

I have been unable to overcome this anger because it makes me feel:

_____

_____

_____

I am still angry about _____

_____

_____

I have been unable to overcome this anger because it makes me feel:

_____

_____

_____

tell you whether it is right or wrong to feel what you are feeling, but rather to support your right to have those feelings. You will be surprised at the amount of relief you experience as you get these feelings off your chest and into the open.

Acting Out Your Angry Feelings

One of the best ways to express your feelings of anger is to literally act them out. Here's how it's done:

- Arrange two chairs facing each other: One is "your" chair, the other is for the person who provoked your angry feelings (a visualized version of him or her). You will use both chairs to act out your feelings.
- Sit in your chair first. Breathe slowly and deeply with your eyes closed until you feel relaxed. Then visualize the target of your anger sitting in the other chair.
- Tell the person in the other chair out loud how you feel. Then stay in your seat and observe how it feels to have said that.
- Now change seats. This time, try to visualize how the other person sees you. Then say out loud what you think this other individual might say to you. When you finish, ask yourself how each of you would feel now.
- Keep changing seats and roles until you have a good idea of how you really feel about the other person and the incident responsible for your anger, and how this individual feels about you. Don't be surprised if you find that your persistent past anger is really due to something different than you thought. And don't be surprised if you discover that the other person is just as hurt and angry as you.

One of the advantages of this technique is that it allows you to vent your feelings to people who are no longer accessible to you for face-to-face communication. Some people find this technique especially helpful for dealing with angry feelings toward a parent who has died or a spouse from a former marriage.

Documenting Your Angry Feelings

Acting out your thoughts and feelings will help you to clarify them greatly. Putting them down on paper will help you to examine them even more carefully. Writing makes them concrete, and puts them in a form that is easier for you to review and evaluate.

A good way to put your feelings down on paper is to write a letter, either to the person who provoked the original anger that is still plaguing you or to yourself. After you have written the letter, reread it several times to be sure that it really reflects what you are feeling and thinking. It is *not* necessary to send the letter to anyone. Just the act of writing helps reduce your level of past anger by helping you to clarify your thoughts and discharge feelings in a nondestructive way.

Making Peace With The Source of Your Angry Feelings

In some cases, it may be appropriate and desirable to actually make contact with the source of your past anger. Any attempt to make contact should be done only if the purpose is to make peace, and there is a reasonable likelihood that the other person shares that goal. Before contacting the other person, you should recognize the risk of failure, and try to imagine how you would feel if that occurred. If you are not sure you could cope with such a failure, do not initiate a peace overture.

If you decide that making peace is a reasonable alternative, here are some things you can do to increase the chances of success:

- Meet the person alone, and take steps to ensure that you are not interrupted.
- Focus on feelings rather than actions. Be honest about what you felt in the past and what you feel now. If you have any positive feelings about the person, express them. Don't be afraid to cry, to laugh, to hug.
- Ask what the other person is feeling. Accept that person's right to have those feelings.
- Tell the person what you would like to see happen as a result of the meeting.

Letting Your Angry Feelings Go

At some point, the best thing you can do is simply let go of your angry feelings. Letting go of them is not the same thing as burying them, but rather a conscious decision that they are taking too high a toll and they are no longer as important as they once were. Sometimes, just saying out loud that your angry feelings are no longer important will help you to put them behind you for good.

As difficult as forgiveness might seem, it can be an important step in letting go of your anger. Forgiving another person does not mean that you condone or excuse their actions, nor will you forget what they've done. But by forgiving them for the wrongs they've committed, you can literally free yourself from your feelings of anger, and rechannel the energy in more productive ways.

Keep in mind that forgiveness is a choice—and a positive choice that can defuse the power of the hurtful events in your past. To move through the process of forgiving, you need to recognize that you have been wronged, but also understand that your resentment may be undermining your own ability to move forward with your life. Instead of hanging onto the grudges and the anger that can take a toll on your physical and mental well-being, forgiveness will allow you to start the healing process, and refocus your emotions in much more positive directions. This process was nicely illustrated in a study at Stanford University that involved young adults who felt hurt or offended by the actions of others. As they were able to genuinely feel and demonstrate forgiveness, their own levels of anger were significantly reduced.

STEP 5: SOLVING YOUR PROBLEMS

Persistent, unsolved problems are common sources of chronic anger. Sometimes problems can go unsolved because they are not correctly identified. Problems also become chronic because there are no practical solutions available. But all too often, problems continue simply because people persist in using ineffective strategies to try to solve them. In other words, the problems are not the problem; the solutions are the problem. There are several ways that solutions become problems:

- When they cannot and do not work, but you persist in trying them

- When they produce short-term success, but create other problems in the long run

- When they create new problems that are worse than the original ones

When your solutions have become the problems themselves, the only way out is to find alternative solutions. The following worksheets will help you find better answers to problems that are sources of chronic anger. Use the worksheets to identify several alternative solutions that might be more successful than the problem-solving strategy you are currently using. Then select the one that seems most likely to succeed, basing your decision on the potential risks and benefits of each. If you need additional worksheets, make photocopies of the ones in the book or use loose sheets of paper to create your own charts.

After you have tried a different approach to a problem, take time to formally evaluate the results. Did your new strategy work better than your old one? If it is not working well, should you return to the old approach, or try one of the other alternatives on your list? These are the questions you should answer yourself every time you use this process.

You should also use this technique for solving new problems. For each new difficulty that arises, identify all of the possible alternative solutions you could try. List why each one might be likely to work or fail. Then write down the risks and benefits of each. Going through this process will increase your chances of selecting a successful solution the first time around, which should result in less angry feelings in the future.

At times, your anger may be provoked by problems or challenges in your life that seem so large, you are literally overwhelmed by them—and by the feelings they generate. In the heat of the moment, you find yourself on the brink of "losing it" completely.

That's when it's essential to take the problem at hand, and break it up into smaller, more manageable parts. Back away from the situation for a brief period, then try to find one small piece of the problem you can focus on, talk about, and—perhaps—solve. This strategy usually will enable you to cope with an anger-provoking problem that otherwise seems overwhelming. It's also a good strategy for cooling off the hot feelings that make it impossible to even think clearly about the problem.

PROBLEM-SOLVING WORKSHEET

1. The problem: _____

_____

_____

2. The solution I have tried: _____

_____

_____

3. Why the solution isn't working: _____

_____

_____

4. Alternative solutions (list, then select best):

a. _____

b. _____

c. _____

5. Potential risks of chosen alternative solution:

_____

_____

6. Potential benefits of chosen alternative solution:

_____

_____

7. Evaluation of results of trying alternative solution:

_____

_____

STEP 6: BUILDING A SUPPORT SYSTEM

Your anger tends to escalate and get out of control when the only person you can talk to about your angry feelings is yourself. To prevent such a situation from occurring, build a support group around you to help you when you become angry. Here are some ways to use a support group:

- Review anger-provoking incidents with the group to get different viewpoints.

- Ventilate your feelings to the group to get them off your chest.

- Enlist the group's advice on how to respond more effectively to anger-provoking situations.

There are important qualities to look for in selecting the people who will form your support group:

- *They should be trustworthy.* Since your angry feelings will often center on personal issues, you cannot afford to share them with someone you don't trust. Choose people who care about you, and who can be relied upon to keep everything you say to them absolutely confidential.

- *They should be competent to help you with the problems you bring to them.* Not every member of your support group will be qualified to help you with all of your problems. So it's a good idea to identify ahead of time what areas of your life you will discuss with whom. For example, it may be very helpful to talk about anger that arises at work with a friend who successfully manages a business, but the same person may not be helpful at all in talking about anger that arises at home.

- *They should be willing to let you make your own decisions.* Getting support from others does not mean letting them direct your life and take over responsibility for your actions. You should not seek support from people who offer it only if you do what they say.

- *They should be willing to help you when you need them.* Sharing someone's angry feelings is not the easiest task in the world, and it is usually not a pleasant one. The people who support you must be willing to put up with a little bit of unpleasantness any time you need them.

Don't forget that the people in your support group may need some support of their own. Make sure they know how appreciative you are for their help, and tell them that you'll be there to help them, too, if they need it.

STEP 7: ANGER MANAGEMENT INTERVENTIONS

Once you've learned to monitor your anger and you've identified your anger triggers, it's time to put the *Anger Management Program* into action. Here are six interventions you can use to manage anger in the future without hurting anyone:

- Counterpunching
- Using anger management statements
- Redirecting your anger in a productive way
- De-escalating your anger
- Developing humor skills
- Using relaxation techniques

Intervention One: Counterpunching

Anger doesn't just change the way you feel, it also affects the way you think. All too often, anger produces distorted thinking that makes the situation worse. These distorted thoughts, or self-statements, then continue the vicious cycle: They produce more bad feelings, which create more distorted thinking.

These distorted thoughts occur very quickly and almost automatically. They are usually very negative, and they are very difficult to turn off. Even though they are usually irrational, we tend to accept these automatic thoughts without even questioning them. In fact, we hardly even notice them when they are occurring, but they exert their negative effect nevertheless.

These distorted thoughts have been likened to mental punches that you throw at yourself. It is important that you learn how to identify these destructive self-statements as soon as they occur and replace them with more productive thoughts. This process is called counterpunching.

There are four different types of distorted thinking that can interfere with the proper resolution of your anger:

- Destructive labeling
- Mind reading
- Magnification
- Imperatives

In the pages that follow, you will learn how to recognize these different types of distorted thoughts when they occur, and you'll identify some appropriate techniques for counterpunching these thoughts.

COUNTERPUNCHING DESTRUCTIVE LABELING

Destructive labeling is the name used when you take a few isolated incidents or observations and generalize them to make an overall negative judgment about someone or something. It always focuses on the negative aspects of any issue or person, and makes you blind to the positive side of things. It creates a continual stream of anger that may be unjust and unnecessary most of the time.

Here's an example of destructive labeling and the kind of counterpunch that must be used to counteract it:

ANGER DISTORTION

Your boss yells at you in front of your colleagues because you forgot to make a sales call that was scheduled. You tell yourself that the boss is an idiot, and you're not going to take any more guff from him.

COUNTERPUNCH

You say to yourself, "I'm really upset that he criticized me in front of all those people. But I actually did screw up, and he doesn't often act that way. He is usually very nice to me so he just must have had a bad day. He wasn't right to yell at me, but it was just one incident."

Now fill in an example of how destructive labeling has distorted your thinking, and identify what you will do in the future to counterpunch when it happens again.

ANGER DISTORTION   **COUNTERPUNCH**

_____   _____

_____   _____

_____   _____

_____   _____

_____   _____

_____   _____

_____   _____

Use a loose sheet of paper to write down all of the other destructive labels you commonly use. Then identify the counterpunch you will use for each in the future.

COUNTERPUNCHING MIND READING

When you try to guess what other people are thinking, you're playing a game called mind reading. You fill in their thoughts, you assign motives to their actions, you even assume what they are feeling. It's alright to play this game, as long as you don't take your guesses too seriously. Once you begin to believe that you know what is on the minds of others, you are setting yourself up for trouble. If it is important that you know what people are thinking, you'll save a lot of time and potential anger by simply asking them.

Here's an example of mind reading and the kind of counterpunch that must be used to counteract it:

ANGER DISTORTION

*You catch your best friend
whispering to another friend.
You assume they are talking
about you. You say to yourself
that your friend thinks you are
vain and silly, even though
she has never said anything
like that to your face.*

COUNTERPUNCH

*You say to yourself, "I don't
really know what they are
whispering about. I'm just
afraid that they're talking
about me. My friend has always
been a good friend who has
treated me with respect and
kindness. I will ask her what
they were whispering about."*

Now fill in an example of how mind reading has distorted your thinking, and identify what you will do in the future to counterpunch when it happens again.

ANGER DISTORTION   **COUNTERPUNCH**

_____   _____

_____   _____

_____   _____

_____   _____

_____   _____

Use a loose sheet of paper to write down all of the other ways in which you commonly engage in mind reading. Then identify the counterpunch you will use for each in the future.

COUNTERPUNCHING MAGNIFICATION

Magnification is the name given to distorted thinking that occurs when you blow something bad totally out of proportion. This kind of thinking can take a relatively unimportant irritant and make it a source of severe and long-lasting anger. You can recognize this form of distorted thinking by the frequent use of words such as *terrible, awful,* and *horrendous.*

Here's an example of magnification and the kind of counterpunch that must be used to counteract it:

ANGER DISTORTION

You get stuck in a traffic jam and you're going to be 15 minutes late for a lunch date. You tell yourself, "This is terrible. My lunch date will be ruined. The day is a total disaster. I can't take this kind of thing anymore."

COUNTERPUNCH

You say to yourself, "Relax. Don't make this situation worse than it is. So I'll be 15 minutes late. That's not the end of the world. If my friend can't understand this delay, it's not my fault."

Now fill in an example of how magnification has distorted your thinking, and identify what you will do in the future to counterpunch when it happens again.

ANGER DISTORTION

_____

_____

_____

_____

_____

_____

_____

COUNTERPUNCH

_____

_____

_____

_____

_____

_____

Use a loose sheet of paper to write down all of the other situations in which you commonly allow magnification to distort your thinking. Then identify the counterpunch you will use for each in the future.

COUNTERPUNCHING IMPERATIVES

Imperatives are inflexible rules that govern the way you act, and the way you think that others should act. You can recognize this form of distorted thinking by the use of such words as *should, ought,* and *must.* You are entitled to set whatever rules you want for your own behavior, but the more rigid they are, the more likely you are to fail to meet them. When you expect others to follow the rules, failure is even more predictable. This failure is bound to lead to anger.

Here's an example of imperative thinking and the kind of counterpunch that must be used to counteract it:

ANGER DISTORTION

Your brother is visiting and helps himself to a snack in the refrigerator. Without saying a word to you, he finishes all of the milk in the house. You are infuriated that he would do this without asking you first whether you wanted some. This violated the rules of etiquette that you follow.

COUNTERPUNCH

You say to yourself, "What's the big deal. He only comes to town twice a year and I love him. Give the guy a break. He hasn't changed in 30 years and I'm not going to change him now. Relax and be more flexible."

Now fill in an example of how imperative thinking has distorted your thinking, and identify what you will do in the future to counterpunch when it happens again.

ANGER DISTORTION

_____

_____

_____

_____

_____

COUNTERPUNCH

_____

_____

_____

_____

_____

Use a loose sheet of paper to write down all of the other situations in which you commonly allow imperatives to distort your thinking. Then identify the counterpunch you will use for each in the future.

Intervention Two: Using Anger Management Statements

One of the most upsetting things about getting angry is that it happens so quickly. By the time you think of an appropriate way to respond, your anger is out of control. In angry situations, an ounce of preparation is worth a pound of cure. That preparation involves creating *Anger Management Statements* that you will use the moment an anger-provoking situation arises.

Here are some *Anger Management Statements* that many people find helpful. Say all of them out loud, and then select the ones with which you feel comfortable. Use them every time you become aware of angry feelings. The sooner you use these *Anger Management Statements*, the better they can work for you.

• Count to ten	• Be patient
• Relax, take a deep breath	• This is not my problem
• Listen, but don't respond	• Sit down quietly, discuss the situation
• Don't take criticisms personally	• Work out an alternative plan
• Stick to the issues	• Be fair
• Don't argue	• Do not yell

In the worksheet that follows, write down your most common anger-provoking situations. Next to each one, list the *Anger Management Statements* you will use to block your anger the next time it occurs (specific instructions that you start saying to yourself the moment you experience any angry feelings). Here is an example:

SAMPLE ANGER MANAGEMENT STATEMENTS WORKSHEET

ANGER-PROVOKING SITUATION

My boss is going to be angry over the way I handled this account. When he calls me in, I know we are going to get into a big argument because he doesn't understand the client and I do. I'll explode because I know I am right.

ANGER MANAGEMENT STATEMENT

I won't yell. I'll take a deep breath and count to ten. I will listen to everything my boss says and I won't take his criticisms personally. I will listen patiently and then try to quietly discuss my point of view and try to work out an alternative plan that includes some of his suggestions.

ANGER MANAGEMENT STATEMENTS WORKSHEET

YOUR ANGER-PROVOKING SITUATION

WHAT STRATEGY WILL YOU USE?

_____   _____

_____   _____

_____   _____

_____   _____

YOUR ANGER-PROVOKING SITUATION

WHAT STRATEGY WILL YOU USE?

_____   _____

_____   _____

_____   _____

_____   _____

YOUR ANGER-PROVOKING SITUATION

WHAT STRATEGY WILL YOU USE?

_____   _____

_____   _____

_____   _____

_____   _____

YOUR ANGER-PROVOKING SITUATION

WHAT STRATEGY WILL YOU USE?

_____   _____

_____   _____

_____   _____

_____   _____

Intervention Three: Redirecting Your Anger in a Productive Way

There are three common styles that people have learned for expressing anger:

- Stuffing
- Escalating
- Directing

Stuffing and escalating are negative ways to express anger. Directing is a positive style.

Stuffing

Stuffing is another term for denial. When you stuff your anger, you avoid the person or the situation provoking your anger. Stuffers pretend they are not upset. They do so because:

- They are afraid of hurting the other person or of being unable to handle the situation themselves.
- They feel guilty or embarrassed about being angry.
- They are afraid of being rejected.

Stuffing sounds like a simple and effective way to avoid angry feelings, but it doesn't work. Stuffed anger breaks out in many different ways, and it can have very serious consequences: It spoils relationships, it harms your health, and it allows your anger to simmer on endlessly.

Escalating

Escalating is a style that attempts to shift the responsibility for an anger-provoking situation to someone else. Escalators accuse others, they swear and they shout.

Escalating doesn't work, because it drives others away. It lets the objects of your anger off the hook—even if your anger is justified—because your behavior is so threatening and offensive. Escalators sometimes win their arguments, but their success is short-lived. Their opponents may give in to avoid ugly confrontations, but in the long run they may try to get even. Escalating destroys relationships and it's bad for your health.

Directing

Directing is a technique that uses anger in a carefully controlled manner to change the condition that is causing the anger. This technique is effective only when another person plays a role in provoking the anger. The technique has three simple steps:

- You reveal the fact that you are feeling angry ("I feel angry...").
- You identify the reason why you are feeling angry ("...because you lied to me...").
- You state the action that the other person could take to eliminate the provocation ("...and I want you to tell me the truth right now, and promise me that you won't lie to me again").

There are many benefits to directing your anger this way: You get your feelings off your chest; you get to the real cause of the problem; you decrease the chances that the same thing will happen again; and your honesty earns the respect of the other person.

However, some people will be very uncomfortable when you try to deal with them directly. These individuals will either avoid your attempts to confront the problem, or they will use techniques to deflect your approach. These techniques are known as "blocking gambits." Commonly used blocking gambits include:

- Making light of your anger by laughing it off or making a joke of it
- Challenging the legitimacy of your complaint
- Blaming you for the problem
- Putting you off until later
- Threatening you or personally attacking you
- Questioning everything you say
- Denying the validity of what you say
- Trying to make you feel guilty

People employ blocking gambits because they feel defensive, and they are afraid to deal with the problem directly. Here are some ways to overcome their blocking gambits:

- Repeat your statements calmly and clearly.
- Point out the fact that the person is avoiding the real issue by using blocking gambits.
- Appear cooperative by acknowledging the person's argument where it is valid, while reiterating your own point of view.
- Refuse to discuss the problem until the other person calms down.
- Ignore threats and get back to the point.

Directing your anger is a much more positive response than stifling it or letting it blow up, but the truth is it won't work all the time, because not everyone responds to this approach favorably. When you can't change the other person's behavior, there's only one thing left to do: Change your own. Whatever you do, don't hold it back or let it get out of control. Pretending you're not angry doesn't work, and stepping up the stakes can lead to disaster.

It's important to be aware of the style you use for dealing with anger. Spend some time thinking about and determining which styles you use the most. You may find that you use one style with some people and a different style with others. Your goal is to learn how to use a direct style with everyone.

Intervention Four: De-Escalating Your Anger

Anger tends to feed on itself and to escalate. This emotional state is likely to occur when two or more people are involved in a confrontation that makes one or both of them feel threatened. Once the escalation process begins, it is difficult—if not impossible—to think and act rationally unless something is done to defuse the situation.

You can defuse the situation by calling *Time Out*. This technique removes you completely from the provocative situation and gives you an opportunity to control the emotional and physical reactions you are experiencing. The procedure for taking a *Time Out* is very simple:

- You let the other person or persons know that your anger is building ("I am beginning to feel very angry...").

- You declare your desire to remove yourself from the situation temporarily ("...and I want to take a Time Out").

- You remove yourself immediately.

Your *Time Out* should last for exactly one hour. Leaving the length open-ended makes it too easy to avoid the problem indefinitely, and also puts other parties at an unfair disadvantage by leaving them in mid-air and at your mercy.

During the *Time Out*, you should try to do something constructive rather than focusing on your anger. Doing something physical such as taking a walk or cleaning out the garage will help you get rid of some of your angry tension. Using relaxation techniques (*Intervention Six*) will help you restore calm to your mind.

After one hour, you should attempt to resume the discussion. A good place to start is by talking about why you called the *Time Out* and how you felt during it. If the other party doesn't want to resume the discussion immediately after the *Time Out*, try to set a mutually agreeable time for talking.

Some anger-provoking situations may be too sensitive to return to in an hour. When that's the case, set another time in the not-too-distant future to deal with the matter. Whatever you do, don't drop the subject and pretend that the anger will go away. Using that approach will just set you up to suffer in the future from past anger.

Intervention Five: Developing Humor Skills

When it comes to dealing with anger, laughter really is one of the best medicines. The more you can learn to laugh at yourself and at some of the things that make you angry, the less trouble you will have with anger in the future. That doesn't mean that you should ignore anger-provoking situations or make light of them. But it is important to keep your life in balance.

Laughter counteracts anger in many ways. It reverses some of the physiological changes that anger causes. Laughter releases the physical and mental tension that tend to maintain anger. Let's face it: It's impossible to feel really angry at the same time you are laughing.

Some people have an innate sense of humor that enables them to find something funny to laugh about at almost any time—even when they are angry. Those of us who lack that ability can—and should—turn temporarily to other laugh-provoking avenues as a way to counter angry feelings. This is one time when sitting down with a humorous book or watching a television comedy program may be good for your health.

Intervention Six: Using Relaxation Techniques

Anger causes muscular tension throughout your body. That tension, in turn, causes emotional and physical discomfort that heightens the unpleasant feelings your anger is causing. You can reverse this cycle by using deep relaxation techniques to calm your mind and release the tension from your muscles.

As you learned in the discussion of stress in Day 3, these techniques alter the way your body reacts to phenomena like anger. You can use these techniques to ease tension and its ill effects, or you can use them in advance of a situation that might provoke anger, thus taking advantage of their preventive properties.

Refer back to Day 3 for descriptions of relaxation techniques that you can use for anger as well as stress. Practice all of them a few times, and then rely on those that work best for you.

A FINAL NOTE

Anger is an unavoidable condition of life—every one of us gets angry at one time or another. We all have different reasons for getting angry, and different ways we react to anger-provoking situations. That's why each of us must create a program specifically tailored to meet our own unique needs, by adapting the seven-step plan outlined in this section. Use the techniques that work well for you, and eliminate the ones that are inappropriate.

Because this program forces you to face some of the things that make you angry, there may be times when using it actually stirs up your anger. Don't let that keep you from using the strategies that can help you learn to manage your anger without hurting yourself or anyone else. With your anger under control, you will find yourself closer to a life of *real* vitality.

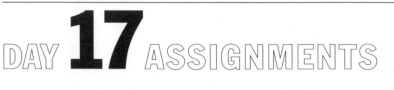 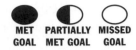

MET GOAL   PARTIALLY MET GOAL   MISSED GOAL

PHYSICAL VITALITY

○ 1. Improve your time for the measured mile by 2 seconds.   **Time**:_____

○ 2. Do all the flexibility and stretching exercises.

○ 3. Do the chest, back and arm strength training exercises.

NUTRITIONAL VITALITY

○ 4. Decrease total fat intake to 10% of total calories.

○ 5. Eat at least 7 half-cup portions of fruits and vegetables.

○ 6. Supplement as necessary to reach the vitamin & mineral recommendations.

○ 7. Limit dietary cholesterol to 300 mg per day.

○ 8. Limit sodium intake to 2,400 mg per day.

○ 9. Consume at least 25 grams of dietary fiber per day.

MENTAL VITALITY

○ 10. Spend at least 10 minutes practicing any deep relaxation technique.

○ 11. Identify and eliminate as many sources of stress in your life as you can.

EMOTIONAL & SPIRITUAL VITALITY

○ 12. If you drink alcoholic beverages, limit your daily intake to one drink if you are a woman or 2 drinks if you are a man.

○ 13. If you do not already volunteer your services, identify one organization in your community that is doing important work, and make a commitment to contribute a significant amount of time within the next two weeks.

MEDICAL VITALITY

SOCIAL CONNECTIONS
AND ALTRUISM   **DAY 17**

Friends and family can be good for your health. A growing number of studies shows that if you have strong and fulfilling relationships, you may live longer, decrease your chances of becoming sick, and cope more successfully when illness strikes. In a landmark report on social isolation, published in *Science* in 1988, Dr. James House and his colleagues wrote that "social isolation is as significant to mortality rates as smoking, high blood pressure, high cholesterol, obesity, and lack of exercise."

Researchers have identified several health issues and medical conditions that are clearly influenced by social isolation. These include:

- **Heart Disease.** Social ties can cut your chances of having a heart attack and reduce other health problems associated with coronary artery disease. In a study reported in the *Journal of the American Medical Association (JAMA)* in 1992, researchers evaluated the impact of social isolation on more than 1,200 people who had already had one heart attack. They found that those individuals who lived alone had nearly a 16 percent likelihood of experiencing a second heart attack (fatal or non-fatal), compared to about 9 percent in those who lived with someone else.

  At the University of Pittsburgh School of Medicine, researchers evaluated the effect that the loss of a partner through divorce can have on the well-being of men. They studied nearly 11,000 men who were married at the start of the study, and who had no evidence of coronary heart disease. After nine years of follow-up, those men whose marriages dissolved had a higher risk of death from a number of causes, including cardiovascular disease. According to the study, published in the *Archives of Internal Medicine* in 2002, those with the greatest mortality risk not only experienced a marital breakup, but also chronic work stress.

- **Stroke.** In 2002, researchers at Columbia-Presbyterian Medical Center reported on a study which found that in people who have already had a stroke, their risk of having a second one was decreased significantly by the number of friends they had, as well as by whether they had in home help. The four-year study of 655 stroke patients concluded that individuals with fewer than four friends were 40 percent more likely to experience a second stroke. Social support was even a greater risk factor than blood pressure, diabetes, gender, marital status, and the presence of a primary-care doctor.

- **Cancer.** In an eighteen-year-long study of more than 6,800 people in Alameda County, California, women participants who had few or no social ties had twice the chance of dying of cancer. Among men who developed cancer, those who had networks of social connections lived much longer than those who were socially isolated. In another study at the Medical College of Wisconsin, unmarried people with cancer had a poorer survival rate than those who were married, even after the researchers took into account the severity of their illness and the type of treatment they received.

- **Immune Disorders.** At Ohio State University College of Medicine, researchers studied the immune systems of 38 married women and an equal number who were divorced or separated. The married women had stronger immune function, and those who reported being happily married had the best immune response, as measured by factors such as the activity of certain disease-fighting white blood cells. (The latter point is particularly significant. It is not enough just to have social connections or to be married. You need to have positive relationships, rather than those caught in the quicksand of conflict. If you have an unhappy marriage, it might actually increase your chances of becoming sick.)

- **Mental Functioning.** At the UCLA School of Medicine, researchers evaluated 1,189 older adults who were active and independent when the study began. After following them for 7.5 years, the investigators reported that those individuals who were in satisfying social relationships when the study began functioned better cognitively at the end of the study, and experienced a slowing of any mental decline. (Surprisingly, those participants who were unmarried had better cognitive abilities over time than their married counterparts; researchers speculated that many married subjects may have done worse because they were caring for an aging spouse.)

In a study in the Netherlands, researchers at Leiden University Medical Center and the University of Amsterdam studied 599 men and women over the age of 85, paying attention to their levels of happiness and contentment with life. Those individuals who were the happiest had incorporated regular social activities into their lives; they tended to have built relationships with friends and family during their younger years. By maintaining those bonds, they were better able to avoid depression, maintain their self-esteem, and remain active as they aged. Even those people who had health-related physical impairments said that these difficulties were of less importance to them than maintaining their social contacts and activities. The lesson to be learned from this: Family and friends can be good medicine.

- **Longevity.** When researchers at the California Department of Health Services and the University of Kuopio in Finland tracked the health of middle-aged men, they found a higher death rate in those men who reported having few sources of social support. By contrast, those who were active in organizations (clubs, churches) had only half the risk of death, compared to those who did not participate in these groups.

Men who perceived the quality of their relationships as poor or "inadequate" had almost twice the risk of death as those with strong social ties. This study demonstrates the importance of nurturing your relationships; it is not just how many people you are connected to, but how well you are connected to them.

- **Nutrition.** Studies also show that men and women who live alone tend to eat less well–to the point that they risk their physical well-being. A study in the *Journal of the American Dietetic Association* in 1990 concluded that men ages 55 and older who lived alone were more likely than married men to eat a diet containing less than two-thirds of the RDAs (Recommended Dietary Allowances) for vitamins A, B_6 and C, and calcium and magnesium. Women living alone also had a greater likelihood of eating vitamin- and mineral-deficient meals.

Unfortunately, modern technology may be pushing us away from forming social ties, rather than fostering them. At the Stanford University Institute for the Quantitative Study of Society, research reported in the year 2000 surveyed 4,113 American adults, questioning them about the effects of Internet use. About 36 percent of the individuals reported being online five or more hours per week, which resulted in significant changes in their lives, including more social isolation. Among these heavy users, about one-quarter said they spent less time with friends and family, and 10 percent spent less time at social events. The researchers noted that "the more hours people use the Internet, the less time they spend with real human beings."

The effect that isolating technologies will have on health status is still not known, but one fact is already abundantly clear: social isolation increases your risk of problems. Here are some suggestions to help you find and nurture social ties:

- Join organizations that appeal to people with interests similar to yours—for example, a group related to your hobbies or political preferences. If you have an illness, find a support group of people with the same health problem.

- Make an effort to contact long-lost friends or family members. Start creating a family tree, for example, and ask close and distant relatives to assist you.

- Seek ways to actively help others. Volunteer at a homeless shelter or a hospital. Become a Big Brother or Big Sister to a fatherless or motherless child. Shovel the snow off an elderly neighbor's driveway. Participate in a fund-raising activity for AIDS or breast-cancer research. Deliver hot meals to senior citizens. Make a financial contribution to your favorite charity.

- Keep track of the amount of time you spend in activities that promote isolation. Set a reasonable daily and weekly limit for yourself, and stick to it.

CAN ALTRUISM KEEP YOU HEALTHY?

As we've pointed out, one way to boost your social connectedness, and improve your own health in the process, is by becoming involved in altruistic, charitable and other worthwhile activities. Some researchers who have studied volunteerism have reported a "helper's high" that comes from showing generosity to others. In research by sociologist Allen Luks, many women volunteers reported experiencing pleasurable physical sensations (feelings of warmth, well-being and calmness, and increased energy levels) both during and after helping other people. They also obtained relief from their own stress-related health problems such as headaches and other aches and pains, and felt a stronger sense of self-worth. Luks theorized that their altruism reduced their own stress levels, which in turn contributed to their physical well-being.

People who have participated in groups such as Alcoholics Anonymous or Overeaters Anonymous know that their own healing process is stimulated by showing concern and compassion to others with similar problems. They form strong connections with others in the group, and that helps create circumstances in which their own well-being can improve.

Here is what other studies on altruism and social support have shown:

- Researchers at the University of Michigan followed more than 2,700 people for over a decade. They found that regular volunteer work had more of a positive effect on life expectancy than any other activity. Men who did *not* participate in volunteer activities had more than twice the chance of dying during the course of the study as those who volunteered at least once a week.

- A landmark study by Dr. David Spiegel at Stanford University evaluated 86 breast-cancer patients who were undergoing traditional medical care, more than half of whom participated in a support group of women with the disease. He found that those who attended the support sessions coped more effectively with their illness, were less anxious and depressed, and had a better quality of life, compared to the group who received only conventional treatment. Dr. Spiegel wrote, "Social isolation was countered by developing strong relations among members.... Clearly, the patients in these groups felt an intense bonding with one another and a sense of acceptance through sharing a common dilemma.... The therapy group patients visited each other in the hospital, wrote poems, and even had a meeting at the home of a dying member."

  The most extraordinary finding came in a follow-up analysis a decade later, which found that women in the support sessions lived an average of 18 months longer than the controls; that represented a *doubling* of survival time. As Dr. Spiegel wrote, "The therapy seemed to influence their bodies' ability to fight back physically."

- A study at the UCLA School of Medicine, published in the *Archives of General Psychiatry* in 1993, reached similar conclusions. Patients with melanoma (a very dangerous cancer of the skin) participated in support group sessions that met for ninety minutes per week for six weeks. Over a period of five years, these participants had a significantly better survival rate than a comparison group who did not take part in a support group; the non-participants had triple the risk of dying from their melanoma than the participants.

Why did these support groups have such a positive effect? Spiegel theorized that these networks not only combat social isolation, but also allow people to feel that they are helping one another. Although we still cannot explain it, this appears to have a positive effect on the body's natural ability to fight disease.

ARE PETS BENEFICIAL TO YOUR HEALTH?

If you're feeling more socially isolated than you'd like to be, your health might get a boost if there is a dog or a cat in your household. People form strong emotional bonds with their pets; these animals are sources of companionship, and are living beings to care for. Pets also show affection and love in return. Studies show that this kind of companionship may promote healing. For example:

- A study at the University of Pennsylvania evaluated more than 90 people who had experienced a heart attack, and followed them for one year after their discharge from a coronary care unit. Those who owned pets had a small but significantly higher survival rate, compared to patients without pets.

- In a study at UCLA, researchers evaluated 345 elderly pet owners and a comparable group without pets. Those with pets needed to visit their doctors less frequently, and pet owners said their animals provided them with comfort in hard and stressful times.

The presence of a pet tends to draw your focus away from yourself and the anxieties in your life, and toward the animal that needs your care and attention. By adopting a pet, you not only obtain a wonderful companion, but you also contribute to your feelings of self-worth and altruism by providing a loving home for an animal.

This approach for dealing with the issue of social isolation may sound simplistic, but research shows that it works extremely well for many people.

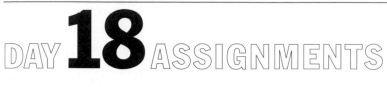

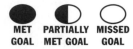

MET   PARTIALLY   MISSED
GOAL   MET GOAL   GOAL

PHYSICAL VITALITY

○   1. Improve your time for the measured mile by 2 seconds.   **Time**:_____
○   2. Do all the flexibility and stretching exercises.
○   3. Do the leg and abdominal strength training exercises.

NUTRITIONAL VITALITY

○   4. Decrease total fat intake to 10% of total calories.
○   5. Eat at least 7 half-cup portions of fruits and vegetables.
○   6. Supplement as necessary to reach the vitamin & mineral recommendations.
○   7. Limit dietary cholesterol to 300 mg per day.
○   8. Limit sodium intake to 2,400 mg per day.
○   9. Consume at least 25 grams of dietary fiber per day.

MENTAL VITALITY

○   10. Spend at least 10 minutes practicing any deep relaxation technique.
○   11. Identify and eliminate as many sources of stress in your life as you can.

EMOTIONAL & SPIRITUAL VITALITY

○   12. If you drink alcoholic beverages, limit your daily intake to one drink if you
are a woman or 2 drinks if you are a man.
○   13. Do Step 1 of *Improving Your Relationships*.

MEDICAL VITALITY

IMPROVING YOUR RELATIONSHIPS

DAY 18

Some people determine the quality of their relationships by the amount of conflict they experience. (*"We never fight, so that means we must have a great relationship."*) But the absence of conflict is no guarantee of a successful relationship (for example, when two partners become so distant from each other that nothing is worth arguing about anymore). Other people measure their relationships by the amount of contact between the partners. (*"We are always together, we talk to each other a lot, we enjoy the same sports, so we must have a great relationship."*) Yet some of the best relationships involve people who are forced by external conditions to remain physically apart for long periods of time. And some of the worst relationships involve people who are constantly together physically, but far apart emotionally. They fight because it feels better than having no contact at all.

Measuring the degree of *connection* between you and your partner is a better way to evaluate the quality of your relationship. Connected partners are interested in each other's thoughts and feelings—especially their feelings about themselves. Connected partners are willing to share these thoughts and feelings with each other, knowing that this information will never be exploited or used against them. Connected partners are still able to maintain their individuality. They can grow and change—even in opposite directions—without jeopardizing their relationship. Indeed, the more they share their changing experiences and feelings, the more the relationship grows, and the closer the partners are drawn together.

This section of the program is designed to help you build closer relationships, and move another step nearer to *real* vitality. The techniques you will learn can significantly improve the quality of your relationships by providing a more effective—and more enjoyable—way to communicate important feelings and needs to the people with whom you are involved. These techniques will help you become more "connected" in your relationships, but you will build closer relationships only if you use them correctly and regularly.

At first, these techniques will feel stilted, artificial and unnatural. That's because they *are* stilted, artificial and unnatural. (The "natural" approach involves criticizing or attacking your partner, and defending yourself.) With practice, it does get easier and feels more natural.

This program works best when both partners are willing to learn and practice the techniques together. But if your partner is unwilling to try the program, use some of these techniques alone. Before long, your partner will begin to respond in a different manner.

STEP 1: TALK, DON'T CRITICIZE

We should be able to solve most relationship problems simply by talking to our partners, but talking often fails to work because so much talk takes the form of criticism. Instead of talking about our own feelings—a step that invites understanding and support—we criticize the behavior of our partner, who then responds by defending, withdrawing or counterattacking. Even our questions can become indirect criticisms if asked in a harsh or demanding tone (*"Why didn't you call me? Where are you going?"*).

Criticism creates conflict, partly because it is judgmental (*"You are bad for doing what you do"*) and partly because every criticism includes a built-in demand for change (*"I don't like the way you do this, so change it"*). But demanding doesn't work, and if you continue criticizing, the only thing that changes is the volume of your arguments. The talking becomes shouting, the dialogue deteriorates into personal attacks, and the partners become defensive. Ultimately, one or both of the partners disconnect from the relationship and withdraw into a shell of silence.

The following conversation shows how relationships can be harmed when talking takes the form of criticism:

LINDA: *This is the third night in a row you've come home late from work!*
DENNIS: *Do you think I like working this hard? I've got a job that keeps me late. What do you expect me to do?*
LINDA: *Well, dinner is cold, the kids are cranky, and I'm about to lose my mind.*
DENNIS: *And I've got a stack of bills to pay—because you don't know how to budget.*
LINDA: *Oh swell, now it's my fault that you're working late. Well, I hope you enjoy your cold dinner alone!*
DENNIS: *I'm not interested in eating anymore. Thanks to you, I've lost my appetite.*

When two partners can't work things out (or even agree on the nature of the problem), it's time to stop working on the problem itself, and move instead to an emotional level—by exploring each other's feelings. This new approach will enable you to understand each other's position and to identify what is interfering with your ability to solve the problem, as well as bring you and your partner closer together.

Be aware that there is a difference between talking about your emotions (such as being angry, sad, happy, anxious) and the feelings you have about yourself (such as feeling incompetent, inadequate or unlovable). It's okay to talk about your emotions, but do not make such talk a substitute for talking about feelings. The only way to achieve intimacy in your relationship is to share your innermost feelings about yourself and give your partner an opportunity to do the same thing with you. Sharing your feelings helps your partner to understand who you *really* are, and to be more supportive of you in the future.

Here's an example of how this might work when a frazzled husband returns home to a frustrated wife:

LINDA: *Thank goodness you're home. I wondered if you had gotten into an accident.*

DENNIS: *I was tied up at work and lost track of the time. Why do you always get so wound up about it?*

LINDA: *Because I get lonely. I even begin to wonder if you still love me.*

DENNIS: *And when you think I don't love you, how does that make you feel?*

LINDA: *Totally unlovable. Frankly, there are days when I wonder why you would love me anyway.*

DENNIS: *I do love you. It's just that I'm overwhelmed at work now. And, frankly, I'm just not feeling very secure about my job. I don't think my boss appreciates anything I do, and I'm afraid of losing my job in the next round of layoffs.*

LINDA: *Oh my. I had no idea you were under so much pressure at work. That must feel awful.*

DENNIS: *It does. To tell the truth, I've never felt this bad. It's as though I've lost all my confidence. I'm actually frightened at times, and that doesn't make me feel very good about myself.*

LINDA: *Is there any way I can help?*

DENNIS: *Just let me get some of this off my chest. It really feels better just to talk about it. And I'll try a little harder to get home earlier.*

Talking about feelings leads to better solutions, because it gets to the real issues that underlie most conflicts and misunderstandings. This kind of talking makes a partner move closer instead of withdrawing or counterattacking. It builds intimacy instead of enmity, and may even change the behaviors that triggered the conflict (like coming home late), although these changes become much less important once the underlying issues are clear.

MANAGING ANGER

If, at any time, you or your partner become too angry to continue talking without being critical or listening without being defensive, stop the discussion and try to talk the angry person down to a calmer state. If this approach doesn't work, or if both partners are too angry to talk, then separate briefly (go into different rooms), and resume the discussion when the anger abates.

Practice Session: Talking Without Criticizing

To begin, schedule a 10-minute talk session during which each partner talks for five minutes while the other partner listens; then change places. Use this session to discuss a specific issue that has created problems in the past. Do not try to solve the problem during this session. Instead, do the following:

While you are the talker:

1. Talk about yourself and how the current situation makes you feel about yourself—not about what your partner does or how you would like your partner to change.
2. Speak in the same manner and tone you would like your partner to use with you.
3. Do not demand or expect anything of the partner who listens.
4. Try not to let yourself become angry (see box: *Managing Anger*, on the previous page).
5. When you are finished talking, ask your partner: *"What did you hear me say?"* If your partner heard something different than what you wanted to communicate, keep talking until you can agree on what has been said.

While you are the listener:

1. Listen carefully to what the talker is saying, and try to understand whatever is said *from the talker's point of view.*
2. Be aware of any statements the talker makes with which you disagree. For the sake of this exercise, accept those statements as true, even if you disagree with them strongly. Try to imagine how *you* would feel if these statements were actually true.
3. Don't judge your partner's feelings. They are neither right nor wrong, but for your partner—they are real.
4. Even if you feel that your partner is criticizing you, do not defend yourself—no matter how much you feel under attack.
5. Try not to let yourself become angry. If either partner becomes too angry to follow these guidelines, stop the session temporarily and resume after things have calmed down (see box: *Managing Anger*, on the previous page).
6. Remain silent whenever silence encourages the talker to continue communicating with you about his or her feelings. If the talker gets "stuck," help out by asking questions, making facilitating statements (*"Oh, that's interesting"*) or offering facilitating instructions (*"Tell me how you feel about that"*). Do not try to solve any problems.
7. Do not switch roles and become the talker until the five minutes are up.

How Did You Do?

After you both had a turn at talking and listening, talk to each other about what you learned from the practice session.

STEP 2: LISTEN, DON'T DEFEND

Listening is one of the most powerful tools you can use to improve your relationships. But many people have difficulty mastering the skill of listening, because they take everything personally and constantly feel the need to defend themselves. They become so preoccupied with defending themselves, they are no longer able to hear anything that is said—except from their own point of view. Their inability to listen makes it impossible for them to hear what their partner is really trying to communicate.

The following conversation illustrates how being defensive can interfere with listening and push partners farther apart:

CHRISTINA: *I feel terrible about what's been happening with us the last few days.*

GREG: *What do you mean?*

CHRISTINA: *We're constantly fighting. You keep telling me that I do things wrong, and you're always yelling at me.*

GREG: *Well, don't blame me for the fights. I'm only trying to be honest with you. And I'm not yelling.*

CHRISTINA: *Yes, you are. You're doing it right now.*

GREG: *Well, you never do anything about my complaints. No wonder I have to yell.*

CHRISTINA: *And you're supposed to be perfect?*

In this discussion, Greg couldn't hear what Christina was trying to tell him because he was too busy defending himself. If Greg had been listening instead of defending, here's how the conversation might have gone:

CHRISTINA: *I feel terrible about what's been happening with us the last few days.*

GREG: *What do you mean?*

CHRISTINA: *We're constantly fighting. You keep telling me that I do things wrong, and you're always yelling at me.*

GREG: *How does that feel when I yell at you?*

CHRISTINA: *It's very frightening. It makes me feel as though I'm a little child. It reminds me of the way my father always screamed at me.*

GREG: *Tell me more.*

CHRISTINA: *I feel as though the only way I can keep you loving me is to simply let you control everything. And that makes me feel like I am going to disappear.*

GREG: *Disappear?*

CHRISTINA: *Yes, it's almost as though the old me would cease to exist. Almost like I was going to die. It's very frightening.*

GREG: *I really didn't mean to make you feel that way, and I'm sorry. Can I talk for a moment about what I'm feeling?*

CHRISTINA: *Please.*

Listening sounds simple, but it's not. In fact, the listener's job is much more difficult than the talker's, because the listener is responsible for keeping the conversation going and for helping the talker to stay focused on feelings. Listening well is also difficult because we tend to hear things from our own psychological point of view instead of the talker's, so we interpret what is said based on our own feelings instead of the talker's. (For example, if we feel incompetent or inadequate, we assume that the talker thinks we are incompetent or inadequate, too.) As a result, we spend too much time defending ourselves unnecessarily, and we withdraw or retaliate. Once you give up the need to defend yourself, your ability to listen is greatly improved, and you find yourself being drawn closer to your partner.

Do not confuse being a good listener with being silent all the time. A good listener asks questions and makes comments when these actions will help the talker to express feelings. But a good listener does not try to get information to satisfy his or her own personal needs or curiosity; it is only for the purpose of understanding the other person.

Here's how you can become a better listener:

1. Be truly interested in the feelings your partner is sharing. Be sensitive about the vulnerable areas or "soft spots" that are being revealed to you.

2. Try to interpret and understand everything from the talker's point of view. Even if you don't agree with what is said, recognize that your partner sees things this way. Try to accept your partner's viewpoint as the truth, and imagine how you would feel if you saw things that way, too.

3. Remain silent until your partner is done talking. Don't interrupt in the middle of a thought or a statement.

4. Practice asking questions that keep the talker focused on feelings, and don't make them complicated (some examples: *How does that make you feel? What is it about that which bothers you? Can you tell me more about that? Is there anything else that could be upsetting you?*). Avoid a questioning tone that is critical or harsh.

5. Practice making facilitating statements and instructions that encourage your partner to continue talking about feelings (some examples: *That's interesting. Tell me more about how you feel and why you feel that way*).

6. Do not try to solve problems or "fix" your partner's feelings. Your only job as a listener is to understand what your partner is saying about himself or herself.

7. Do not take any of your partner's comments personally, and don't attempt to defend yourself against anything that is said.

8. When you are done, try to reach agreement about what the talker has said.

Practice Session: Listening Without Defending

Schedule a 10-minute talk session during which each partner talks for five minutes while the other partner listens; then change places. Use this session to discuss a specific issue that has created problems in the past.

While you are the listener:

1. Try to understand whatever is said *from the talker's point of view.*

2. Be aware of any statements the talker makes with which you disagree. For the sake of this exercise, accept those statements as true, even if you disagree with them strongly. Try to imagine how *you* would feel if these statements were actually true.

3. Don't judge your partners feelings. For your partner—they are real.

4. Do not defend yourself—*no matter how much you feel under attack.*

5. Try not to let yourself become angry. If either partner becomes too angry to follow these guidelines, stop the session temporarily and resume after things have calmed down (see box: *Managing Anger*, page 177).

6. Remain silent whenever silence encourages the talker to continue communicating with you about his or her feelings.

7. If the talker gets "stuck," help out by asking questions, making facilitating statements (*"Oh, that's interesting"*) or offering facilitating instructions (*"Tell me how you feel about that"*). Do not use your comments as an attempt to solve any problems.

8. Do not switch roles and become the talker until the five minutes are up.

While you are the talker:

1. Talk about yourself and how the current situation makes you feel about yourself—not about what your partner does or how you would like your partner to change.

2. Speak in the same manner and tone you would like your partner to use with you.

3. Do not demand or expect anything of the partner who listens.

4. Try not to let yourself become angry (see box: *Managing Anger*, page 177).

5. When you are finished talking, ask your partner: *"What did you hear me say?"* If your partner heard something different than what you wanted to communicate, keep talking until you can agree on what has been said.

How Did You Do?

After you both had a turn at talking and listening, talk to each other about what you learned from the practice session.

STEP 3: GET BENEATH THE SURFACE

The arguments of most couples tend to focus on issues like money or in-laws or who is responsible for certain tasks around the house. Although these issues can seem very important at the time the arguments are taking place, in reality they are really surface issues or "red herrings." If these relatively minor (or at least manageable) problems were the only issues, the arguments would be over very quickly. After all, it's not that difficult for two people to figure out how much money they have and how to spend it, or to decide whose job it is to do which tasks around the house. These surface issues are rarely the real problems; unless the real problems are addressed, the arguments will go on forever.

When couples argue endlessly over seemingly insignificant matters, the real issues usually have to do with unresolved problems from childhood or with control. (The partners are really arguing at an unconscious level about who is in charge of the relationship.)

There are two sides to the control issue: The fear of being enveloped or swallowed up (*"How much of myself do I have to give up to be in a relationship with you?"*) and the fear of abandonment (*"If I give myself up to you, what guarantee do I have that you will not hurt me or leave me?"*). But these fears are never limited to just one of the partners. Once couples recognize that both partners fear being controlled, and both are struggling and defending their positions, they can take steps to become advocates for each other, rather than being adversaries.

The following conversation illustrates how focusing on surface issues can obscure the real problems that lie beneath:

MARCIA: *I made reservations for us to go to New York for our vacation.*

DAN: *How could you do that? I don't want to go to New York.*

MARCIA: *We always vacation where you want to go. This year, we're going to New York because that's where I want to go.*

DAN: *In fact, last year we vacationed with your parents. This year, it's my turn to choose! We're going camping in the Grand Canyon!*

MARCIA: *You know that I hate camping.*

DAN: *Well, for a change, do what I want. It's only fair, Marcia.*

How can two people see the same facts so differently? Because this argument has nothing to do with facts. The issue of where to go on vacation is a surface issue that could be solved in 60 seconds. For example, how about this negotiated settlement: *"From now on, I'll choose the vacation spot in even-numbered years and you'll choose it in the odd-numbered years."* The real issue for this couple is about control—or about feeling controlled.

How do you get to the real issues that lie beneath the surface? By talking and listening to each other about feelings instead of focusing on behaviors. Instead of arguing about who earned the money and who spent it, talk about how money (or the lack of it) makes you feel. Instead of arguing about who did which task and who didn't, talk about what task-sharing means to you, how you feel when tasks aren't done, and why you feel that way.

Here's how Dan and Marcia could have ended their argument quickly—by talking about feelings instead of focusing on the surface issue:

MARCIA: *I made reservations for us to go to New York for our vacation.*

DAN: *How could you do that? I don't want to go to New York.*

MARCIA: *Why are you so upset that I want to go to New York?*

DAN: *Because you didn't even ask what I thought of the idea. You seem to automatically expect that we'll go there.*

MARCIA: *And how does that make you feel?*

DAN: *It feels bad. It's like my opinion doesn't even count. Even worse.*

MARCIA: *What do you mean?*

DAN: *It makes me feel as though I don't count—not just my opinions. And that hurts.*

Whenever you and your partner are in conflict over an issue that should easily be settled, you're almost certainly arguing about a surface issue and missing the real problem beneath. Once you identify the real issues—by talking about feelings— the surface issues will disappear and your conflict will end. This process will also bring you and your partner closer together.

Practice Session: Getting Beneath the Surface

Sit down with your partner and work on a seemingly superficial problem that crops up again and again and creates conflict in your relationship. Then ask each other the following questions:

1. What feelings does this issue trigger for you?
2. Why do you think this issue triggers those feelings?
3. Can you identify another time in your past when a similar issue triggered such feelings, or can you recall a different issue in your past that triggered similar feelings?
4. Why does this issue trigger such feelings now?

Take turns talking and listening to each other's answers until you believe the real underlying problem is defined. Then make another attempt to deal with the surface issue in a manner that leaves you both feeling more comfortable.

How Did You Do?

After you have each taken several turns talking and listening, talk to each other about what you learned from the practice session.

STEP 4: BEWARE OF "THE VOICE BEHIND"

Whenever you have a strong emotional reaction to something your partner says or does, you must consider the possibility you are reacting to something other than what was actually said or done. You may be reacting instead to feelings from the past that have been "stirred up" or "triggered" by current events. Such a reaction is especially likely if the intensity of your feelings seems far out of proportion to what your partner has said or done.

We call this reaction "responding to the voice behind," because it's a reaction to your past feelings and experiences, not to the person in front of you. In someone whose parents were constantly critical, a benign comment or criticism can trigger a flood of angry emotions. And a well-meaning offer of assistance can trigger the same reaction from someone whose parents controlled every aspect of his or her childhood. Responding to the voice behind is a common reaction in anyone who has unresolved issues and conflicts from earlier in life (which means all of us).

The following conversation illustrates how the "the voice behind" can disrupt communication and distance partners from each other:

CINDY: *Well, what do you think of my paint job in the kitchen?*

BILL: *You did a great job, but I'm a little disappointed with the color. It's a little darker than I thought it would be.*

CINDY: *What do you mean?*

BILL: *I wanted just a little lighter shade of blue.*

CINDY: (exploding) *Well, that's gratitude for you. Next time, paint it yourself.*

BILL: *Why are you so upset? All I said was that I thought we had picked a lighter color.*

CINDY: *I'm fed up with you putting down everything I do. I'm just sick of it!*

BILL: *Well, I'm sick of you getting so upset over nothing. What's wrong with you? I'm going for a walk.*

Why did Cindy go into such a rage? Because she grew up with a mother who was overly critical of everything she did. When Bill criticized the color of the kitchen paint, he became Cindy's mother for a few moments, triggering all of the old feelings of worthlessness and anger. Cindy heard her mother talking (the voice behind) and reacted to Bill's comments with the same emotions and reactions that her mother had sparked when she was young. Of course, Bill responded by getting angry as well. A simple issue, like the color of paint, started a major argument that distanced this couple further from each other.

How could Bill and Cindy have dealt with this issue in a better manner? The following conversation illustrates a healthier approach:

CINDY: *Well, what do you think of my paint job in the kitchen?*

BILL: *You did a great job, but I'm a little disappointed with the color. It's a little darker than I thought it would be.*

CINDY: *What do you mean?*

BILL: *I wanted just a little lighter shade of blue.*

CINDY: (exploding) *Well, that's gratitude for you. Next time, paint it yourself.*

BILL: *Cindy, what's going on? Why is my opinion about the color of the kitchen making you so upset?*

CINDY: *I don't know.*

BILL: *What are you feeling? Let's sit down and talk about it.*

CINDY: *Bill, I feel like I can never do anything right. That's what my mother told me when I was young. She belittled everything I did. It seems that I did everything wrong.*

BILL: *And how did that make you feel?*

CINDY: *Totally worthless. And that's the way I felt when you criticized the color I painted the kitchen. Worthless.*

BILL: *I didn't mean my comment about the color as a criticism of you. Don't forget—I'm the one who picked that color. And I'm getting more fond of it by the moment. You did a great job. I don't see a single brush stroke.*

CINDY: (giggling) *That's because I used a roller.*

You can't stop feelings from the past from breaking through once in a while, but you can keep them from inappropriately influencing your behavior today, and you can prevent them from interfering with your relationship. To gain control of these feelings, you and your partner must recognize when the voice behind is "speaking" and learn to respond to it in a different manner. Mastering this task will prevent many serious arguments and promote greater closeness in your relationship.

Practice Session: Recognizing "The Voice Behind"

With your partner, identify a small issue that triggered a reaction that seemed out of proportion to the problem. Talk about the feelings that caused your tempers to flare, and try to link those feelings to your past experiences (the voice behind). Ask your partner:

1. What memories or old feelings did the recent experience rekindle?
2. Who did I represent from your past?
3. Where were you when you last experienced feelings like this?
4. How will you recognize voices from your past when they return again?
5. How can I help you deal with "voices from the past"?

How Did You Do?

Talk to your partner about what you have learned from this session.

STEP 5: DON'T TAKE RESPONSIBILITY FOR YOUR PARTNER'S FEELINGS

Understanding and accepting how your partner feels about himself or herself is a critical step toward achieving a close and intimate relationship and being truly "connected." But some people try to go beyond understanding and acceptance to the point where they feel *responsible* for their partner's feelings. They need to "fix" things so their partner will feel good, so they give suggestions, provide direction and make demands—in essence, taking control of their partner's life. Some do this because it makes them anxious to do nothing when their partner is suffering, others do it because they need to control everything in their relationship. Whatever the reason, the process is extremely damaging to the relationship.

The following conversation illustrates how one partner's attempts to "fix" things for the other partner can backfire:

CHERYL: *Hi, honey, how was your day?*

JAY: *Terrible. I've been feeling very depressed since we moved to this city, and I'm not sure what to do about it.*

CHERYL: *You've really got to try to snap out of this. How about the new suits you got last weekend? I thought that would put you in a better mood.*

JAY: *I guess it didn't.*

CHERYL: *Well, I don't know what else to do. I've sent flowers. I bought gifts. I've done everything I know to cheer you up, and I'm at the end of my rope. It's beginning to make me angry that you're so depressed all the time! What else can I do?*

It's no surprise that both partners would feel worse after an exchange like that. Cheryl tried to take responsibility for how Jay felt, when all he really wanted her to do was to listen and to accept his feelings without judgment. That acceptance would have given him comfort.

In a good relationship, partners are not responsible for each other's feelings. When one partner is sad or depressed, it is not the other partner's job to create happiness. It's an impossible task that is doomed to fail, and that failure will only make the "fixing" partner feel frustrated, more anxious and—ultimately—angry. The most comforting thing any partner can do for another is to listen attentively, be completely accepting, and be responsive to any specific requests that are made (*"Hold me"* or *"Just let me talk"*).

Imagine how both Jay and Cheryl might have felt if the following conversation had taken place instead:

CHERYL: *Hi, honey, how was your day?*

JAY: *Terrible. I've been feeling very depressed since we moved to this city, and I'm not sure what to do about it.*

CHERYL: *Tell me what you're depressed about.*

JAY: *It's just so lonely for me here, Cheryl. I feel like I'm starting all over, and that it's going to be such a monumental effort to meet people and make new friends.*

CHERYL: *I'm really sorry you're in this situation. It must be a little frightening. Tell me what you are feeling.*

JAY: *I am scared. I'm afraid I won't be able to pull myself out of this mood. I feel just like I did when I was a kid and my family moved to Los Angeles.*

CHERYL: *Why is it so upsetting for you to move?*

JAY: *My father ran out on the family shortly afterward. And I guess I'm just feeling a bit insecure with you now.*

CHERYL: *How did you feel when your father ran out on you?*

JAY: *I was not good enough. I felt like it was my fault. I felt like I was a bad person.*

CHERYL: *It wasn't your fault, and I am not your father. And I really love you, and I'll try to support you in any way I can. Is there anything I can do now?*

JAY: *For now, just hold me.*

It's not possible to "fix" the way another person feels. So, what can you do if you still feel responsible for your partner's feelings? Learn how to be responsive to them instead. Learn what your partner is feeling and why. It isn't necessary to change anything. There is enormous healing power in your willingness to simply accept feelings as they are.

Practice Session: Accepting Feelings

Talk to your partner about the way the two of you deal with feelings. Ask each other the following questions:

1. Do you feel free to share all feelings with me?
2. Do you actually share all of your feelings? If so, talk about the last time you did it, and discuss how you felt afterward.
3. If you do not share feelings, what is it that keeps you from doing so?
4. How do you really feel about yourself?
5. Are there any specific needs I can meet for you, without having to take responsibility for the way you feel? (In response, be very specific. Avoid answers like *"Help me feel better about myself,"* because those requests are impossible to fulfill. Make requests that the other person can actually respond to, like: *"Hold me," "Take me for a walk,"* or *"Come home at the time you say you're going to."*)

How Did You Do?

Talk with your partner about what you learned from this session.

TIPS AND TRAPS
Closing The Distance

It seems logical that all couples would try to form the closest bond possible. In reality, most couples do the opposite: They work hard to maintain a comfortable distance between themselves. Why? Because getting too close to another person—revealing too many inner secrets and trusting too much—leaves you vulnerable to being hurt.

Most couples avoid this danger by creating an emotional (and sometimes physical) distance. In some couples, it's a great distance; in others, it's short. But once the distance is agreed upon, it's usually defended strongly. If one partner tries to close the gap by sharing feelings, the other partner almost instinctively backs away by withdrawing, or starting an argument, or simply becoming too busy with other activities. Barriers go up, and the couples return to the old patterns that helped them maintain a comfortable distance.

The distance can be closed if the partners begin to share feelings about themselves (not just their good feelings, but also their fears and feelings of inadequacy, incompetence and vulnerability). Sharing these feelings enables your partner to understand who you really are, and moves the relationship to a deeper level.

Changing Your Partner

Most people believe that their relationship would improve if they could just get their partner to change. It's wishful thinking, because it is not possible to make someone change. In fact, the more you try, the more the other person is likely to harden his or her position, and the more the relationship will suffer.

Change is much more likely if your partner *wants* it to occur. How do you make that happen? There are three steps to the process:

1. First, give up trying to change your partner. Once you stop trying to force change, your partner is free to move closer to you.
2. You must become more interested than ever in your partner. Be willing to listen as your partner talks. As that happens, your partner may begin to see aspects of his or her behavior that could be improved with change.
3. Talk more about yourself with your partner—especially how you feel about yourself. Do you feel insecure, inadequate, undesirable? These are your "soft spots"—areas of vulnerability. Once you are willing to reveal weaknesses, a loving partner will stop picking on them. The changes you could never *force* in your partner will begin to happen *voluntarily.*

Solving Problems, Resolving Conflicts

It's not possible to have meaningful relationships without experiencing some problems and disagreements between the partners. The goal is to manage these issues in a way that avoids serious conflict.

There are three primary ways to solve problems and resolve disagreements: through control, bargaining, or empathy. When control is used to solve problems, one partner simply dictates the solution to the other. This approach gets the problem solved quickly, but creates a much larger problem because of the resentment and anger the controlled partner will feel. Bargaining is a better way to solve problems, because it can produce a fair solution through the process of compromise. But the empathic approach is even better—especially if you can't resolve the issue through bargaining.

The first step in the empathic approach is to stop trying to solve the problem. Instead, share the feelings you're experiencing because of the issue (don't confuse *emotions* like anger or anxiety with *feelings* such as incompetence or inadequacy). Talking about these feelings makes it possible to identify the deeper issues that are interfering with your ability to solve the problem. It also helps you find a solution that will meet the most important needs of both partners without either partner feeling "put upon" or controlled. The empathic approach not only solves problems, but also brings partners closer together.

Reaching Perceptual Agreement

The term "perceptual agreement" means simply that both partners have agreed upon a reality (in other words, they are talking about the same thing). Such an agreement can happen even if the partners don't agree on the facts of the situation, as long as one of the partners is willing to accept the other partner's perception—even just temporarily—so a meaningful discussion can take place.

Perceptual *dis*agreements happen all the time. For example, two people can perceive the same sunny, cloudless day quite differently; One sees it as "perfect", while the other person (who is depressed) sees it as a "dreadful" day. If they argue about what kind of day it is, there will be no end to the conflict because the day is, in fact, perfect for the first person and dreadful for the second, and no amount of arguing will change that.

The first step in resolving a perceptual disagreement is getting each partner to recognize that—no matter what the *facts* are—each partner's perception *feels* real to that partner. The next step (a much harder one) is trying to see things from the other partner's point of view; it means temporarily accepting the notion that the other partner's perception is the correct one.

It's difficult to adopt your partner's different perception of things if you strongly believe that yours is the correct one. But the goal of this process is not to be correct, but *connected*, and the only way to do that is by truly understanding what your partner is feeling. If both partners are willing to try to resolve a conflict in this manner, the conflict will rapidly evaporate.

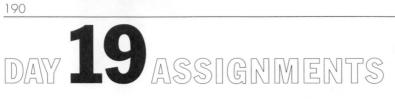

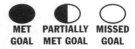

MET GOAL   **PARTIALLY MET GOAL**   **MISSED GOAL**

PHYSICAL VITALITY

1. Improve your time for the measured mile by 2 seconds.   **Time:**_____

2. Do all the flexibility and stretching exercises.

NUTRITIONAL VITALITY

3. Decrease total fat intake to 10% of total calories.

4. Eat at least 7 half-cup portions of fruits and vegetables.

5. Supplement as necessary to reach the vitamin & mineral recommendations.

6. Limit dietary cholesterol to 300 mg per day.

7. Limit sodium intake to 2,400 mg per day.

8. Consume at least 25 grams of dietary fiber per day.

MENTAL VITALITY

9. Spend at least 10 minutes practicing any deep relaxation technique.

10. Identify and eliminate as many sources of stress in your life as you can.

EMOTIONAL & SPIRITUAL VITALITY

11. If you drink alcoholic beverages, limit your daily intake to one drink if you are a woman or 2 drinks if you are a man.

12. Do Step 2 of *Improving Your Relationships*.

13. Do the questionnaire and exercises in this section of the book.

MEDICAL VITALITY

SETTING
PRIORITIES   DAY 19

If you found out today that you had only four more weeks to live, would you live them the same way you spent the past four weeks (or any typical four weeks) of your life? Many people are upset by that question—not because the thought of death frightens them, but because they've spent so much of their lives pursuing things that seem unimportant when time is running out. Large homes, fancy cars, high salaries and prestigious jobs aren't so attractive when you're not around to enjoy them.

If you learned that your time on Earth was now suddenly very limited, would you be able to say that all of your priorities had been in the right place? Would the people around you—especially your family and friends—agree? It's time to start asking these questions now.

What does setting priorities have to do with vitality? Everything—when you define vitality in its fullest sense. Jogging a mile in seven minutes won't create *real* vitality if you dread going to work every morning. Lowering your blood pressure or your cholesterol level won't result in *real* vitality if there's a growing distance between you and your loved ones. And consuming vitamins and minerals in optimal doses doesn't produce vitality if you've put your spiritual needs on the back burner.

Setting priorities and living your life by them is an essential step toward achieving *real* vitality. It's also the best way to ensure that your life is continuously filled with pleasure and fulfillment instead of stress and disappointment. People who set inappropriate priorities (particularly those who spend all of their time and expend all of their energy at the workplace) often end up feeling stressed and anxious or depressed. They wake up to the need for changing priorities only when a crisis arises—the threat of a divorce, the unexpected death of a favorite relative or friend, or their own development of a life-threatening illness.

The shocking events of September 11, 2001, increased everyone's awareness about the fragility and unpredictability of life. In the aftermath of that event, as the victims were memorialized, the importance of setting priorities—and respecting them—became painfully clear. Many families took solace from the knowledge that they were the top priority in the lives of their now-lost loved ones. Others were left wishing—too late—that the priorities in their family had been different.

Don't wait for a crisis to occur in your life or in the world before you reevaluate your priorities. Now is the time to rethink and redefine the meaning of personal "success," and reconsider how you will spend the future. Today's assignments will help you reevaluate your life.

EVALUATING YOUR CURRENT PRIORITIES

The first assignment for today is to evaluate your current priorities.

1. If you found out today that you had only four more weeks to live, would you live them the same way you spent the past four weeks (or any typical four weeks) of your life?   ○ YES   ○ NO

2. Has your focus on career success, money and material objects been appropriate and in balance with the rest of your life?   ○ YES   ○ NO

3. Have all of your priorities been in the right place?   ○ YES   ○ NO

4. Would your family and friends agree with the answers you gave to questions 2 and 3?   ○ YES   ○ NO

5. In the left-hand column, rank the following common priorities according to the amount of time, attention and energy you actually dedicated to them during the last four weeks (be careful not to confuse your desired behavior with the way you actually lived your life during this period). Rank each item on the list from 1 to 10 (with the highest priority receiving a "1" and the lowest getting a "10").

Rank During Past 4 Weeks	*Priorities*	*Rank During Next 4 Weeks*
_____	*Work hard for promotions, salary increases*	_____
_____	*Achieve status in the eyes of your peers*	_____
_____	*Accumulate wealth*	_____
_____	*Collect material possessions*	_____
_____	*Improve your health*	_____
_____	*Improve your relationship with your spouse or loved one*	_____
_____	*Spend time with your children*	_____
_____	*Make time for personal enjoyment*	_____
_____	*Spend more time with friends*	_____
_____	*Tend to your spiritual needs*	_____

Once you have settled on a final ranking, it's time to ask yourself this critical question: If you had only four more weeks to live, would you follow the same priorities and live your life the same way you did during the last four weeks? If your answer to this question is "yes," your assignment for the day is over. If the answer is "no," or if you have any uncertainty about the answer, re-rank your priorities according to the importance you think they should have during the next four weeks. As you prepare this new and "ideal" list of priorities, don't let practical issues interfere with your ranking. Although some circumstances in your life may make your most important priorities more difficult to achieve, you should not use that as an excuse to remove them from the list or to downgrade their importance. Doing that will only decrease your likelihood of achieving the ideal.

If you're having trouble completing this exercise, consider asking for some help from family and friends. Getting their reaction can be especially helpful if you believe that many of your current priorities are based on meeting the needs of others instead of your own (more often than not, this belief turns out to be an elaborate rationalization for continuing your old behavior). And don't be afraid to think about changing the status quo. Recognizing that you're working too hard and ignoring family priorities doesn't mean you have to quit your job—but there's nothing wrong with thinking about that option.

Finally, it's time to ask the most important question of all: What are you going to change in the next four weeks (and the rest of your life) to bring your actual behavior in line with the priorities you have set for yourself? If you don't answer this question thoughtfully—and in a practical way—you risk spending more of your precious time chasing priorities that will have little meaning in the future. It really doesn't matter if the next four weeks of your life are the last. You only get one chance to live them, so live them well.

In the space on page 194, write down the changes you will make to bring your actual behavior more in line with the priorities you have said were most important to you. Make your entries as specific and practical as possible, so they can be monitored and measured in the days to come. For example:

If your priority is to spend more time with your children, you might write:

I'll come home for dinner every evening, and spend time asking each of my children about his or her day. I'll also set aside part of every evening to help the kids with their homework, or at least review it after they've completed it.

If work is consuming nearly all of your time—at the expense of your other important priorities—you might write:

I will talk to my boss tomorrow about restructuring my job. If that takes me off the fast track to another promotion, I will accept that as the price of living a more fulfilling personal life.

If you are not taking any time for personal enjoyment or growth, you might write:

I will read one novel a week. I will take an art class at night to improve my painting skills. I will call some old friends whom I haven't spoken to in years.

In the space below, write down the changes you will make over the next four weeks to align your behavior with your priorities.

CHANGES THAT I WILL MAKE

1. _____

_____

2. _____

_____

3. _____

_____

4. _____

_____

5. _____

_____

6. _____

_____

7. _____

_____

8. _____

_____

SOME FINAL THOUGHTS ABOUT PRIORITIES

The tragic events of September 11, 2001, made all to clear the unpredictability of life. Reevaluating your priorities should be a continual process in *your* life. Every four weeks, repeat the exercises described above—reviewing the priorities you set for the past four weeks, asking yourself if you really lived by those priorities, and resetting your priorities for the next four weeks. If one of your priorities no longer seems quite as important as before, move it down your list or replace it with a new priority that has more meaning. Setting priorities on a regular basis will make your life more meaningful—and more fun.

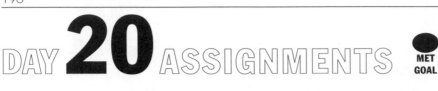

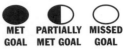

PHYSICAL VITALITY

○ 1. Improve your time for the measured mile by 2 seconds.   **Time:**_____
○ 2. Do all the flexibility and stretching exercises.
○ 3. Do the chest, back and arm strength training exercises.

NUTRITIONAL VITALITY

○ 4. Decrease total fat intake to 10% of total calories.
○ 5. Eat at least 7 half-cup portions of fruits and vegetables.
○ 6. Supplement as necessary to reach the vitamin & mineral recommendations.
○ 7. Limit dietary cholesterol to 300 mg per day.
○ 8. Limit sodium intake to 2,400 mg per day.
○ 9. Consume at least 25 grams of dietary fiber per day.

MENTAL VITALITY

○ 10. Spend at least 10 minutes practicing any deep relaxation technique.
○ 11. Identify and eliminate as many sources of stress in your life as you can.

EMOTIONAL & SPIRITUAL VITALITY

○ 12. If you drink alcoholic beverages, limit your daily intake to one drink if you
     are a woman or 2 drinks if you are a man.
○ 13. Do Step 3 of *Improving Your Relationships*.
○ 14. Answer this question: "If you learned that you had only one month to live,
     would you change the way you spent this day?"

MEDICAL VITALITY

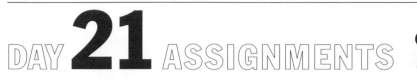

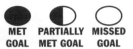

MET GOAL   PARTIALLY MET GOAL   MISSED GOAL

PHYSICAL VITALITY

○ 1. Improve your time for the measured mile by 2 seconds.   **Time:**_____

○ 2. Do all the flexibility and stretching exercises.

○ 3. Do the leg and abdominal strength training exercises.

NUTRITIONAL VITALITY

○ 4. Decrease total fat intake to 10% of total calories.

○ 5. Eat at least 7 half-cup portions of fruits and vegetables.

○ 6. Supplement as necessary to reach the vitamin & mineral recommendations.

○ 7. Limit dietary cholesterol to 300 mg per day.

○ 8. Limit sodium intake to 2,400 mg per day.

○ 9. Consume at least 25 grams of dietary fiber per day.

MENTAL VITALITY

○ 10. Spend at least 10 minutes practicing any deep relaxation technique.

○ 11. Identify and eliminate as many sources of stress in your life as you can.

EMOTIONAL & SPIRITUAL VITALITY

○ 12. If you drink alcoholic beverages, limit your daily intake to one drink if you are a woman or 2 drinks if you are a man.

○ 13. Do Step 4 of *Improving Your Relationships*.

○ 14. Answer this question: "If you learned that you had only one month to live, would you change the way you spent this day?"

MEDICAL VITALITY

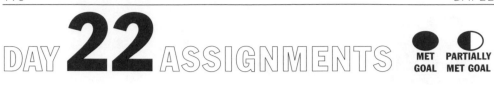

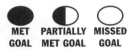
PHYSICAL VITALITY

- ◯ 1. Improve your time for the measured mile by 2 seconds.   **Time:**_____
- ◯ 2. Do all the flexibility and stretching exercises.

NUTRITIONAL VITALITY

- ◯ 3. Decrease total fat intake to 10% of total calories.
- ◯ 4. Eat at least 7 half-cup portions of fruits and vegetables.
- ◯ 5. Supplement as necessary to reach the vitamin & mineral recommendations.
- ◯ 6. Limit dietary cholesterol to 300 mg per day.
- ◯ 7. Limit sodium intake to 2,400 mg per day.
- ◯ 8. Consume at least 25 grams of dietary fiber per day.

MENTAL VITALITY

- ◯ 9. Spend at least 10 minutes practicing any deep relaxation technique.
- ◯ 10. Identify and eliminate as many sources of stress in your life as you can.
- ◯ 11. If you did not awaken this morning feeling rested, refreshed and looking forward to the day, make a commitment to increase the amount of time you sleep tonight by at least an hour.

EMOTIONAL & SPIRITUAL VITALITY

- ◯ 12. If you drink alcoholic beverages, limit your daily intake to one drink if you are a woman or 2 drinks if you are a man.
- ◯ 13. Do Step 5 of *Improving Your Relationships*.
- ◯ 14. Answer this question: "If you learned that you had only one month to live, would you change the way you spent this day?"

MEDICAL VITALITY

HOW TO GET A GOOD NIGHT'S SLEEP

DAY 22

Did you spend last night tossing and turning? Did you desperately but futilely try to find a comfortable position—from your back to your stomach to your side—that might finally send you off to sleep? When the alarm clock finally buzzed this morning, did you stumble out of bed, dazed and irritable, wondering how you would make it through the day?

Well, you're not alone. Insomnia affects one-third of all adults in the U.S. When you're sleep-deprived, your ability to concentrate, your job performance, and your decision-making skills decline a few notches (just ask a hospital intern whose long shift hasn't permitted him or her any sleep). People who are short on sleep also suffer from headaches and mood swings, and their risk of workplace and automobile accidents rises.

If your insomnia is a chronic problem, it can also impair your overall physical health. Poor sleep may increase your susceptibility to illnesses (including colds and sore throats) by weakening your disease-fighting immune system. The body uses sleep to recharge and rebalance certain physiological processes, although researchers still cannot tell us precisely how the body does it.

Researchers have discovered that a good night's sleep is fairly complicated. It consists of repeated cycles during which we go from light sleep to deep sleep and back to light sleep again. Each full cycle lasts about ninety minutes and consists of several stages. During stages 1 and 2, slumber is very light—so light, in fact, that people who spend the whole night in these stages due to sleep disruptions may say, "I didn't sleep a wink all night." Individuals who feel the most rested after a night of sleep are those who spend plenty of time in stages 3 and 4—the deepest stages—during their ninety-minute cycles. There is also a stage of sleep called "REM" (which stands for rapid eye movement), during which the brain is extremely active, dreaming occurs, and the eyes dart rapidly under closed eyelids. Some researchers believe that, to feel well-rested the next morning, we need to pass through an average of four complete cycles of sleep per night.

HOW MUCH SLEEP DO YOU NEED?

You know you've had enough sleep when you awaken in the morning without the help of an alarm clock, and feel alert and rested during the day. Most of us require seven to eight hours of *good* sleep *every* night to feel this way. When we don't get it, we suffer (often, the people around us suffer, too).

But not everyone needs the same amount of sleep. Some individuals actually get only three to four hours of sleep per night—and thrive! Others struggle through the day if they don't get nine or ten. Thomas Edison and Winston Churchill got by quite well on only four hours (although they catnapped occasionally during the day); by contrast, the *New York Times* has reported that one college professor required 14 hours per night, or he would feel groggy and anxious the next day.

WHAT KEEPS US AWAKE?

Your ability to get a good night's sleep can be disrupted for a variety of reasons. The anxiety associated with the illness or death of a family member or a close friend may cause you to toss and turn. Worries about work deadlines, the loss of a job, money problems, your child's school difficulties, or an argument with your spouse also can keep you from getting enough sleep. (A recent study at the University of California, San Francisco, concluded that family concerns and responsibilities are the primary reasons why women under age 40 can't sleep.) Or imagine trying to sleep with the all-night pain that some medical conditions cause. Some stimulant medications can keep you awake, too, as can depression and other psychiatric problems. And once these conditions have kept you up for a few nights, your worries about not sleeping can cause more anxiety that turns your sleeplessness into a chronic problem, even after the initial cause has been resolved.

Women may have some unique sleep difficulties. Pregnant women are often awakened during the night by an increased need to urinate or by the discomfort of their changing body shape. During menopause, the discomfort associated with hot flashes can cause insomnia. (A study at the University of Washington in Seattle found that 23 percent of menopausal women experienced sleep difficulties.) Hot flashes occurring at night may awaken some women 20 to 30 times per night, and could be responsible for the daytime fatigue and irritability that some women experience.

STRATEGIES FOR SLUMBER

To achieve *real* vitality, you must get all the sleep your body needs. Even if you don't suffer from chronic insomnia, you may still need more sleep than you're getting now. The following techniques can help:

- **Adopt a regular sleep schedule.** Your body has an internal biological clock that regulates your periods of sleepiness and wakefulness. If your body is "scheduled" to fall asleep at 10:30, it will probably be difficult to doze off at 9:30 instead. To synchronize your body with its internal clock, try to get up at the same time each morning (even on weekends), no matter how well or how poorly you've slept. Go to bed only when you're feeling sleepy. Don't work against your biological clock.

- **Choose your time for exercise carefully.** Regular, vigorous exercise helps most people sleep better. However, if you work out too close to bedtime (within two to three hours before you get under the covers), it may actually keep you awake. Exercise can raise your body temperature and adrenaline levels, and stimulate your mind—not the best state to be in for sound sleep.

  If you can exercise only in the evening, do so early so your body temperature will fall by the time you're ready for sleep. In a recent study at Virginia Commonwealth University, people who stopped exercising in the late evening cut the time it took them to fall asleep by 22 minutes. In research at Johns Hopkins University, volunteers who exercised earlier in the day experienced improvements in the length and quality of their sleep.

  Of course, if you're fatigued from a chronic lack of sleep, exercise may be the last thing you feel like doing. But if you take a mile walk about three hours before retiring for the night, you may never have those rundown feelings again.

- **Avoid stimulants such as caffeine and nicotine in the hours before bedtime.** Many people don't drink coffee late in the day, but overlook the fact that many teas and soft drinks contain caffeine; there is even caffeine in some over-the-counter medications— including certain cold preparations, pain-relievers, and allergy drugs. Chocolate contains a chemical like caffeine that acts like a stimulant. And if you smoke—quit. Smokers spend less time in deep and REM sleep, because of the nicotine they inhale.

- **Keep away from stressful activities.** For at least a couple of hours before getting into bed, don't ruminate about the rat race at work, stay away from the stack of unpaid bills, and avoid confrontations and arguments with your spouse. If you're thinking about things you need to do tomorrow, put them down on paper so you can get them off your mind. Spend the late evening hours listening to your favorite music, reading a good novel, or watching television. However, avoid late-night TV chillers or action-packed books. If you begin a great mystery novel just before bedtime, you may not be able to put it down until you finish.

- **Select your "midnight snacks" carefully.** Eat only small amounts of food before bedtime—and choose them carefully. Your stomach doesn't stop digesting just because you've gone to bed, and the rumbling stomach from a big meal can keep you awake. Avoid spicy foods that can cause indigestion. Better choices are a glass of warm milk or protein-rich foods like turkey, beans or cheese, which contain an amino acid called tryptophan; this substance promotes the production of a brain chemical called serotonin, which helps induce sleep. (While tryptophan was once available in pill form in health food stores, that is no longer the case.)

- **Become a teetotaler.** A drink before bed may actually help you doze off more quickly (a recent national survey of people with sleep difficulties found nearly 30 percent of them rely on alcohol to help them get to sleep). But don't count on alcohol keeping you asleep. As alcohol is metabolized, mild withdrawal symptoms can actually upset your sleep mechanisms and cause restlessness for the rest of the night. People who use alcohol to get themselves to sleep are more likely to have bleary eyes in the morning.

- **Play soothing music at night.** When you get into bed, turn on a nearby clock radio to some relaxing music that can help put you to sleep. Set it to shut off after 30 minutes. Find other ways to relax in bed, too. Try relaxation exercises after you get into bed (see the information in Day 3 for examples of these techniques). Or take a hot bath shortly before bedtime. A long, hot shower or bath can also help relieve any aches and pains you may be feeling, and this will make it easier to fall asleep.

- **Don't take naps.** If you feel tired during the day, go for a brisk ten-minute walk rather than catching a few winks on the couch. A nap will undermine your need for sleep that night. One man went to the beach for a week's vacation, dozed on the sand, took a nap before dinner, and then wondered why he had trouble sleeping at night.

- **Don't fight it.** If you can't sleep, don't make the situation worse by worrying about how tired you're going to be in the morning, and don't try to "force" yourself to sleep. Instead, get out of bed and read, or write a letter to a friend, or watch TV (pick the most boring program you can find!). Lie down again only when you feel sleepy.

  Also, don't use your bed for anything other than sleep (sexual activity is the only exception to this rule). Don't read in bed, work on your laptop computer, pay bills, eat, or watch TV. You shouldn't associate your bed with anything other than sleep and relaxed feelings. Make sure your bedroom is dark, quiet, and neither too hot nor too cold (a temperature of 60 to 65 degrees is comfortable for most people).

TRY REPETITIVE ACTION

Many people are helped by a relaxation and "unstressing" technique called repetitive action. By concentrating your thoughts *totally* on the repetition of a single sound, sight, or act, your body will relax enough to allow sleep to take over. Practice it at bedtime for a few nights, and see what happens. Here are a few examples of how repetitive action works:

1. **Rock-a-bye.** Lay your head on the pillow and very gently rock it from side to side. Concentrate totally on the motion of your head. The first few nights, it may take a few minutes before the movement lulls you to sleep. With practice, you can condition yourself so well that just a few nods will be all it takes to make you doze off.

2. **Use repetitive imagery.** Gather an imaginary flock of animals on one side of a fence and start them jumping over one at a time, counting them as they go. Yes, it's the old counting-sheep trick—but it works for many people. If you think sheep are a bit old hat, use cats, dogs, deer, or any other animals that make you sleepy. Don't stop counting until you're asleep. Over the course of time, you'll be counting less and sleeping more.

3. **Try counting backward.** Beginning with the number 1,000, start counting downward . . . 999, 998, and so on. Say each number silently to yourself, and at the same time, create a visual image of each numeral in your mind. The first time you use this technique, you may have to recite several hundred numbers before you doze off. The more you use this technique, however, the faster it works. Some people who use it regularly report that they are never able to get below 900 before falling asleep.

WHEN TO CALL THE DOCTOR

If your sleep difficulties become chronic, see your doctor to be sure that you do not have a serious disorder such as sleep apnea, or another medical problem that is keeping you awake. If your doctor can't solve the problem, consider visiting a specialized sleep-disorders clinic, with a staff skilled at pinpointing and resolving your sleep difficulties.

Some doctors prescribe sleeping pills, but I think they should be used only in rare instances. While these pills may put you to sleep, they often won't allow you to spend enough time in the deep stages of sleep, nor to dream as much as normal, both of which are essential for health. Regular users of these drugs frequently develop a dependence and even a tolerance to them, requiring larger and larger doses to achieve the same effect. Once you stop taking sleeping pills, the return of normal dreaming can actually cause "rebound nightmares." Then the pills can become the problem instead of the solution.

The only time sleeping pills may make sense is in response to an extremely stressful situation in your life. For example, if you can't sleep due to the death of a loved one, using these drugs for a few days may be worthwhile.

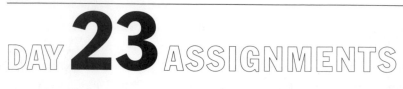

DAY 23 ASSIGNMENTS

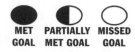

MET GOAL   PARTIALLY MET GOAL   MISSED GOAL

PHYSICAL VITALITY

1. Improve your time for the measured mile by 2 seconds.   **Time:_____**
2. Do all the flexibility and stretching exercises.
3. Do the chest, back and arm strength training exercises.

NUTRITIONAL VITALITY

4. Decrease total fat intake to 10% of total calories.
5. Eat at least 7 half-cup portions of fruits and vegetables.
6. Supplement as necessary to reach the vitamin & mineral recommendations.
7. Limit dietary cholesterol to 300 mg per day.
8. Limit sodium intake to 2,400 mg per day.
9. Consume at least 25 grams of dietary fiber per day.

MENTAL VITALITY

10. Spend at least 10 minutes practicing any deep relaxation technique.
11. Identify and eliminate as many sources of stress in your life as you can.
12. If you did not awaken this morning feeling rested, refreshed and looking forward to the day, make a commitment to increase the amount of time you sleep tonight by at least an hour.

EMOTIONAL & SPIRITUAL VITALITY

13. If you drink alcoholic beverages, limit your daily intake to one drink if you are a woman or 2 drinks if you are a man.
14. Answer this question: "If you learned that you had only one month to live, would you change the way you spent this day?"

MEDICAL VITALITY

15. Review the screening guidelines. Call your doctor to discuss any tests you might need based on the guidelines described in this section.

SCREENING TESTS

DAY 23

Screening is a way to identify medical problems in their very earliest stages, at a time when they are most easily treated, and when it is most likely that serious problems can be prevented. For example, routine Pap smears enable physicians to detect and treat abnormalities on the cervix before cervical cancer develops, and blood cholesterol tests can help identify people at high risk for coronary heart disease, most of whom can reduce their risk by making simple dietary changes. Another form of screening is a routine physical exam. Even though you may feel perfectly healthy, the exam gives your doctor an opportunity to find problems before they cause any symptoms.

The idea of regular screening first got a big lift in 1922, when the AMA proposed the concept of annual physical examinations—even for people who were healthy. The idea caught on quickly and gradually expanded over the next few decades to include other kinds of screening procedures, including blood tests, urine tests and chest x-rays. Special laboratories and businesses sprang up just to promote screening, some offering to perform 24 tests or more on a single specimen of blood. It wasn't long before some doctors were ordering these tests on all of their patients at every visit. It was certainly good for business, but how good was it for the patients? The answer: Not necessarily good for their health, and especially not good for their pocketbooks.

The truth is that you need to choose your screening tests carefully; you can get too much of a good thing. There are direct risks associated with some screening tests, ranging from painful bruising after a needlestick to an increased rate of cancer from excessive chest or dental x-rays. And there are the risks and costs related to inaccurate test results. No test is perfect, so for every thousand performed, you've got to assume that some will incorrectly come out negative (meaning they will fail to diagnose a problem that is present), and some will incorrectly come out positive (meaning they will diagnose a problem that doesn't exist). In the first case, you won't be at any more risk than if you hadn't had the screening test, although the erroneous test result can give you a false sense of security and keep you from seeking therapy when you need it. But the latter case—what doctors refer to as a "false positive" result—can start you down an expensive and risky path of further unnecessary testing. A false positive Pap test report may lead to a biopsy of the cervix, and a false positive test for blood in the stool may lead to telescopic and x-ray examinations of your colon. These procedures are not justified when they are triggered by an inaccurate screening test.

Another problem with some screening tests is that—even though they may detect some problems earlier—they don't always change the final outcome. One example of this is the use of routine pelvic ultrasound tests to screen women for ovarian cancer. The cure rates are no higher for women whose cancers are found this way than for women whose cancers are found during routine pelvic exams. Another example of this problem involves the use of chest x-rays to screen for lung cancer. By the time a lesion is large enough to appear on an x-ray, it's too large to be treated any more effectively than a cancer that's detected after symptoms (usually a cough) arise. So screening the entire population with chest x-rays doesn't improve the cure rate for those who develop lung cancer.

The best approach to screening (as with almost everything else in health care) is to balance the potential risks against the potential benefits. When a screening test offers a good chance of detecting a problem early enough to make a difference in the way you will be treated or in the outcome of that treatment, and when the test has a high degree of accuracy and a low level of associated risks and cost, it makes sense to get it. When the opposite is true, you are wasting your time and money, and exposing yourself to unnecessary risk.

For example, if you are 30 years old and in perfect health, getting an electro-cardiogram to screen for heart disease does not make sense. And a screening test for HIV infection is worthless if you're in a mutually monogamous relationship, you don't use IV drugs and you've never had a blood transfusion.

Deciding which screening tests to have would be much easier if there were a single set of guidelines that all doctors followed. Unfortunately, no such overall set exists. In fact, different sets of guidelines have sprung up for some individual tests, so doctors will differ in their recommendations about which screening tests you should have, depending on which guidelines they choose to follow.

In some cases, you may be helped in making your decisions about screening tests by the recommendations of reputable organizations like the American Cancer Society, the American College of Obstetricians and Gynecologists or the National Cancer Institute. For example, these organizations have now agreed on uniform guidelines for Pap test screening. If you are in doubt about a screening procedure your doctor is recommending, consider contacting a national health organization that deals with that particular issue. (To locate the phone numbers or addresses of an organization, call the reference librarian at your local library or call 1-800-555-1212 to see if the organization has a toll-free number.)

Another source for information on screening guidelines is a book called *Guide To Clinical Preventive Services*, which is a report by the U.S. Preventive Services Task Force. (Note: The book is written in rather technical language, since it was intended primarily for use by health care professionals.) In 1996, this Task Force released its report evaluating the effectiveness of a variety of screening tests and other health-related preventive services; revisions of some of the recommendations were issued in 2001. In developing its reports, the Task Force reviewed scientific literature and research to determine what the real costs, risks and benefits were for each test and service, and it made recommendations about which tests and preventive services are justified on a routine basis, and which are not.

As you review the screening test guidelines that follow you will note that The Task Force recommendations do not necessarily coincide with the guidelines that other groups such as the American Cancer Society are making, and which many physicians are following. For example, if a screening test exists for a particular disease, but there are no medical therapies available to cure or treat that disease, the Task Force usually recommends against screening. In this section, you will find a summary of the Task Force's recommendations. Where these recommendations conflict significantly with those of other major medical organizations, we have tried to identify the difference.

You can use the screening guidelines that follow as a starting point for discussing screening tests and preventive services with your physician. If your doctor recommends a screening test that the Task Force has concluded is unnecessary or not cost-effective, you should ask your doctor to explain why the test is appropriate in your particular case. Keep in mind that the Task Force recommendations apply to the population at large. Based on your personal medical history and/or physical examination, your doctor may be aware of certain circumstances that justify the use of a particular test or service in your individual case.

Read all of the guidelines that follow to learn which ones are applicable to you, and to determine if any action is needed in your case to conform with the recommendations or to clarify your situation. In either case, put a large "X" across the oval next to the screening test as a reminder to talk to your doctor about that test.

SCREENING FOR HEART DISEASE
Blood Pressure   Action Needed ◯

Blood pressure should be measured regularly in everyone aged twenty-one and over. The pressure should be measured at least once every two years if the last pressure readings were below 140 systolic and 85 diastolic. If the last diastolic blood pressure was between 85 and 89, the pressure should be measured annually. Higher readings require more frequent blood pressure measurements. Hypertension (high blood pressure) should not be diagnosed on the basis of one blood pressure measurement. Elevated pressure readings should be confirmed by multiple measurements at each of three separate visits.

Cholesterol Screening   Action Needed ◯

The most recent report of the National Cholesterol Education Program, released in 2001, recommends that all adults twenty years of age and older have a "lipoprotein profile" every five years. This profile measures total cholesterol, LDL cholesterol, HDL cholesterol, and triglycerides (blood drawing for these tests should be preceded by a twelve-hour fast). If a fasting lipoprotein profile can't be performed, the NCEP recommends that total cholesterol and HDL cholesterol levels be measured; if the total cholesterol is 200 mg/dl or higher, or the HDL cholesterol is below 40 mg/dl, a follow-up lipoprotein profile should then be ordered to measure LDL cholesterol and triglyceride levels.

Depending on the outcome of these tests—and whether you already have evidence of coronary heart disease and/or its risk factors—your doctor may recommend other tests and provide additional guidance and treatment.

Electrocardiograms (also known as EKGs or ECGs)   Action Needed ○

This test measures the electrical activity of your heart, which can tell your doctor if your heart rhythm is normal and may reveal if your heart muscle has been damaged previously by a heart attack. Routine screening electrocardiograms are not advised for adolescents or young adults, nor are they recommended for middle-aged and elderly adults, unless they have symptoms that suggest heart disease. Screening electrocardiograms may be advisable in adults who are free of symptoms if either of the following conditions applies:

- Multiple risk factors for coronary heart disease (see box below), if the results would influence treatment decisions

- It would endanger public safety if they had a sudden heart attack (for example, pilots)

The American Academy of Family Physicians recommends a baseline EKG for men 40 years and older if they have two or more cardiac risk factors, as well as for men who have been sedentary and are planning to begin a vigorous exercise program.

RISK FACTORS FOR CORONARY HEART DISEASE

- High blood pressure

- Current cigarette smoking

- Family history of coronary artery disease (heart attack or sudden death before age 55 in a male parent or sibling, or before age 65 in a female parent or sibling)

- Male sex (over age 45)

- Female sex (over age 55, or with premature menopause without estrogen replacement therapy)

- Low HDL cholesterol (HDL less than 35, confirmed by repeat measurement)

- Non-insulin-dependent diabetes

SCREENING FOR DIABETES   Action Needed ⭕

Diabetes is a condition that causes the blood glucose (sugar) level to rise. If untreated, the abnormally high glucose levels increase the risk of cardiovascular disease, stroke, kidney disease, blindness and many other problems. However, long before these complications occur, the abnormal sugar levels will cause symptoms that should alert physicians to measure blood glucose levels. Therefore, routine screening for diabetes in men and nonpregnant women is not recommended but may be considered in selected high-risk groups, including:

- Obese individuals (20 percent or more over ideal weight) over age 40

- Ethnic groups, including Native Americans, African Americans, and Hispanics

- People with a family history of diabetes

- Women at risk for diabetes during pregnancy (gestational diabetes), due to factors such as obesity and older maternal age

SCREENING FOR THYROID DISEASE (OTHER THAN CANCER)   Action Needed ⭕

The thyroid gland plays an essential role in regulating metabolism in the body (the rate at which your body creates and uses energy). Thyroid hormones also influence many other processes and organs throughout the body. When the thyroid gland is producing excessive amounts of hormone (hyperthyroidism), many symptoms and physical changes can develop, including restlessness, irritability, insomnia, heat intolerance, shortness of breath, diarrhea, weakness, shakiness, rapid heart rate, weight loss and bulging of the eyes. When the gland produces too little hormone (hypothyroidism), the symptoms and physical changes can include confusion, memory loss, weight gain, constipation, hair loss, shortness of breath, numbness, lethargy and inability to tolerate cold temperatures. All of the symptoms listed above can be caused by conditions other than thyroid disease, which explains why the diagnosis is often missed or delayed.

The diagnosis of thyroid disorders is usually made by means of blood tests. These tests are very useful in people who have the symptoms noted above, because they help to distinguish those who have thyroid disorders from those who have other problems. The American Thyroid Association recommends that adults be screened for thyroid dysfunction by measurement of serum thyrotropin concentration (a blood test), beginning at age 35 and every 5 years thereafter. More frequent testing may be appropriate for anyone who has symptoms that might be caused by thyroid dysfunction and for individual at high risk for developing thyroid disease (postpartum women, the elderly and individuals with Down's syndrome).

SCREENING FOR ANEMIA   Action Needed ◯

Anemia is a disorder related to red blood cells, which are responsible for carrying oxygen throughout the body. In people with anemia, the oxygen-carrying capacity of the blood is decreased because there are too few red blood cells or because their ability to carry oxygen is impaired. There are several different causes of anemia, including hemorrhage (bleeding), iron deficiency and heredity.

Anemia is diagnosed by measuring the number of red cells that are present in a blood specimen or by measuring the amount of hemoglobin present in the red cells. In the past, many physicians performed these blood tests routinely as part of an overall examination. However, studies show that this type of screening is rarely helpful when performed in healthy people. Therefore, these tests should be done only when there are symptoms or physical signs that suggest the possibility that anemia is present (pale skin, rapid pulse, lethargy, shortness of breath), or when there is reason to believe that a person has lost substantial amounts of blood.

The American College of Obstetricians and Gynecologists recommends routinely testing pregnant women for anemia at their first prenatal visit and again early in their third trimester.

SCREENING FOR BACTERIA IN THE URINE   Action Needed ◯

In most cases of urinary tract infection, there will be symptoms (fever, frequent urination, pain or burning on urination). However, it is possible for a urinary infection to occur without symptoms, especially in pregnant women, obese individuals, diabetics and the elderly.

The most accurate procedure for detecting bacteria in the urine is a culture test, but this test is time-consuming and expensive. Therefore, most clinicians use a "dipstick" test (a chemically treated paper strip is dipped into the urine specimen; if bacteria are present, the paper strip should change color). If this dipstick test is positive, a urine culture must be performed to identify exactly which type of bacteria is present (this is done by keeping a specimen of urine warm in an incubator for a day or two to promote growth of any bacteria that are present).

The Preventive Services Task Force does not recommend the routine screening of adolescents or adults, but advises all pregnant women to be screened at least once (at 12-to-16 weeks gestation) for bacteria in the urine (more often if a physician believes there are other reasons to suspect that bacteria may be present). The American Academy of Family Physicians, however, recommends screening all people at high risk, including: the morbidly obese, individuals with diabetes, women with a history of gestational diabetes, and all men and women ages 65 and older.

SCREENING FOR OSTEOPOROSIS
Bone Density Measurements   Action Needed ◯

Osteoporosis is a condition in which the bones lose excessive amounts of calcium and thus become more brittle and susceptible to fracture. Among the contributing factors to osteoporosis are calcium deficiency, hereditary susceptibility, lack of estrogen, smoking and sedentary lifestyle. The problem is much more common in women after menopause, when estrogen levels decline (this hormone prevents the loss of calcium from bone).

It is possible to screen for osteoporosis or reduced bone density using x-rays of the bone to determine if calcium is being lost. However, routine testing in healthy women is not recommended. It may be justified around the time of menopause in women who are at high risk for osteoporosis to help determine if hormone replacement therapy is appropriate. The following are considered risk factors for osteoporosis:

- Caucasian or Asian

- Small size (less than 5'2" tall, weighing less than 105 pounds) or fair skin

- A family history of osteoporosis

- Smoker or long history of prior smoking

- Sedentary lifestyle

- Early removal of the ovaries (before menopause)

- An inadequate consumption of calcium in the diet

- Intake of excessive amounts of caffeine or alcohol

SCREENING FOR BREAST CANCER
Breast Examination   Action Needed ◯

The American Cancer Society advises an annual clinical breast exam every three years between ages 20 and 39, and then an annual exam starting at age 40; the American Academy of Family Physicians recommends these exams by a health professional every one to three years for women ages 30 to 39, and annually starting at age 40.

Mammography   Action Needed ◯

Mammography uses x-rays to identify early signs of breast cancer—before a lump can be felt. Mammography should only be done by experienced radiologists in facilities that have been certified by the American College of Radiology. This is the best way to ensure that you are getting the lowest possible radiation dose, and that the mammograms will be interpreted by a qualified physician.

The Preventive Services Task Force recommends mammography every one to two years for all women beginning at age 50 and continuing until age 69. However, the National Cancer Institute recommends mammograms every one to two years starting at age 40. These guidelines differ somewhat from those of the American Cancer Society, which recommends a mammogram every year beginning at age 40. Other organizations agree that, particularly in women at high risk for breast cancer because of their family history, annual mammography may be a good idea from age 40 on. Mammography may also be indicated at any age if a woman has breast-related symptoms or abnormalities in the breast on physical examination.

SCREENING FOR CERVICAL CANCER
Pap Exams   Action Needed ◯

The Pap smear is obtained by gently scraping cells away from the surface of the cervix. These cells are placed on a glass slide and then examined under a microscope for signs of cancer or precancerous changes. If precancerous changes are detected and the cervix is treated, it is possible to prevent the later development of cancer.

Regular Pap exams are recommended for all women who are (or who have been) sexually active, and who have a cervix. Testing should begin at the age a woman first engages in sexual intercourse or at age 18, whichever comes first. Pap tests should be performed at least every three years, although according to the American Cancer Society, the test should be conducted annually until three consecutive annual tests are normal. Thereafter, a three-year interval between Pap exams may be appropriate. A physician may recommend more frequent Pap tests if a woman has any of the following risk factors for cervical cancer:

- Early onset of sexual intercourse

- A history of multiple sexual partners

- Low socioeconomic status

Pap tests may be discontinued at age 65, but only if previous tests have been consistently normal.

SCREENING FOR PROSTATE CANCER   Action Needed ◯

Prostate cancer is the most common cancer in men. The risk of prostate cancer increases with age, beginning around the age of 50 (although, rarely, it does occur earlier). In its earliest stages, while the cancer is still confined to the prostate gland, it rarely produces symptoms. The primary screening tests for diagnosing prostate cancer are the digital rectal exam and the PSA (prostate specific antigen) blood test. During the digital rectal exam, the physician feels the prostate through the rectum for signs of enlargement, lumps, or abnormal hardness. The PSA test looks for increased amounts of a protein that is often manufactured at greater levels when prostate cancer is present.

The Preventive Services Task Force does not recommend routine screening for prostate cancer. The American Cancer Society, however, recommends screening by digital rectal exam and PSA as indicated below.

Digital Rectal Exam   Action Needed ○

The American Cancer Society recommends that a digital rectal examination be performed annually beginning at age 50 in all men with a life expectancy of at least 10 years. Men at high risk (including those of African decent or those with a first-degree relative diagnosed at a younger age) should begin testing at age 45.

Prostate Specific Antigen (PSA)   Action Needed ○

The American Cancer Society recommends that men age 50 and older have a yearly blood test to check levels of prostate specific antigen (PSA); PSA screening can start at age 40 for African-American men, and those with a family history of prostate cancer. The Task Force's "non-recommendation" is based in part on the fact that the PSA test is not always accurate; many men without prostate cancer will have elevated PSA levels, leading to unnecessary concern and, in some cases, unnecessary biopsies of their prostate gland.

SCREENING FOR TESTICULAR CANCER   Action Needed ○

Testicular cancer most commonly occurs between the ages of 20 and 35. However, men of any age should seek prompt medical attention if they develop any worrisome symptoms such as testicular pain, swelling or heaviness.

Although the Preventive Services Task Force makes no recommendations about routine testicular screening in men without symptoms, it recommends that men at increased risk of developing testicular cancer be told about the availability of screening. These include men with a history of any of the following:

- A testicle that did not descend fully into the scrotum during gestation

- A testicle that has atrophied (become smaller)

- An operation to attach the testicle to the scrotum (orchiopexy)

The American Cancer Society advises a cancer checkup that includes a testicular exam every three years after age 20, and annually after age 40.

SCREENING FOR COLORECTAL CANCER

Colon cancer is the fourth most common cancer in the United States. The long-term survival rate is much better in those who are diagnosed early than for those in whom the cancer is found in later stages.

The primary screening tests for colon cancer include digital rectal examination, fecal occult blood testing and sigmoidoscopy. Rectal examination may detect tumors at the end of the colon, but it cannot identify the presence of any tumors beyond the reach of the examining finger. To examine beyond that point, your doctor must use an instrument (sigmoidoscope or colonoscope) that permits visual examination of the interior surface of the colon. This test is uncomfortable, time-consuming, and expensive. Fecal occult blood testing is based on the fact that colon cancers may cause small amounts of bleeding to occur, even very early in the development of the tumors. Although there may be too little blood present in the stool to visualize with the naked eye, it is possible to detect very tiny amounts with a simple chemical test that your doctor can perform in the office on a stool specimen.

Digital Rectal Examination   Action Needed ○

This procedure should be a part of every complete physical examination your physician performs.

Occult (Hidden) Blood Testing   Action Needed ○

Testing the stool for hidden blood is controversial, since it has been difficult to prove that this procedure increases the cure rate for colorectal cancer. However, a recent study has demonstrated that the death rate from colon cancer can be cut by 33 percent if the screening test for hidden blood is performed every year. (In people who were tested every two years, there was no reduction in overall mortality.) The American Cancer Society recommends that as one option for colorectal cancer screening, stool occult blood testing can be conducted annually, beginning at age 50.

The start of screening at an earlier age may be appropriate for individuals at particularly high risk for colon cancer, including:

- Those who have a parent or sibling who had colon cancer

- Women who have had cancer of the endometrium (the lining of the uterus), or of the breast or ovary

- People who have previously been diagnosed as having inflammatory bowel disease (ileitis or colitis), adenomatous polyps of the colon or colorectal cancer

Sigmoidoscopy Action Needed ○

Periodic flexibile sigmoidoscopy (examination of the interior of the colon through a special viewing instrument) is recommended by the American Cancer Society every five years, starting at age 50, as one option for colorectal cancer screening. The Task Force recommends a sigmoidoscopy every three to five years beginning at age 50, but was unable to determine if sigmoidoscopy is preferable to occult blood testing, or whether a combination of the two is best.

The American Cancer Society also advises a colonscopy every 10 years, starting at age 50, as another alternative for colorectal cancer screening.

SCREENING FOR LUNG CANCER Action Needed ○

Cancer of the lung is the leading cause of cancer deaths in the United States. In the past, screening for lung cancer has been done by examining chest x-rays and sputum cytology specimens (this involves microscopically examining cells from the surface of the breathing tubes that are coughed up with sputum). However, there is little evidence that screening for lung cancer this way reduces the mortality from this disease. Therefore, routine screening for lung cancer is not recommended by either the Task Force or the American Cancer Society.

SCREENING FOR SKIN CANCER Action Needed ○

Skin cancer is the most common cancer in the United States (more than 800,000 new cases are diagnosed every year). Although skin cancers are easily treated and highly curable when diagnosed early, they can be very disfiguring and even life-threatening when allowed to progress (skin cancer accounts for about 9,600 deaths per year).

The principal screening test for skin cancer is physical examination of the skin. You can perform this test yourself in front of a full-length mirror, looking for the following: any change in the color, size or shape of a mole, or sores or lesions that crust, bleed or fail to heal. The American Cancer Society recommends a skin examination by a physician every three years between ages 20 to 39, and annually at age 40 and over, as part of an overall cancer-related check-up.

SCREENING FOR OVARIAN CANCER

Although not one of the most common cancers, ovarian cancer is among the most lethal in women, accounting for nearly 14,000 deaths per year. The primary screening tests for ovarian cancer include pelvic examination by a health professional, blood testing for CA-125 (a protein that is increased in some patients with ovarian cancer) and ultrasound examination of the pelvis. None of these procedures is very accurate for making the diagnosis of ovarian cancer.

Pelvic Examination   Action Needed ◯

A pelvic exam can reveal when an ovary is enlarged, but other procedures—usually involving surgery—are necessary to determine if the enlargement is due to cancer or the result of a benign process. The American College of Obstetricians and Gynecologists and the American Cancer Society recommend an annual pelvic examination, which includes examination of the ovaries. (Note: Pap tests are not necessarily done at every exam).

CA-125 Blood Test   Action Needed ◯

This test is not recommended for routine screening because of its low level of accuracy. The CA-125 level can be abnormally high in people without cancer or in women with benign (noncancerous) problems of the ovaries. Also, it can be normal in women who have ovarian cancer.

Pelvic Ultrasound   Action Needed ◯

This test is not recommended for routine screening because it is expensive and has a low level of accuracy. Ultrasound testing produces false positive results in a significant percentage of women with healthy ovaries, leading them to undergo additional testing that is risky, expensive and unnecessary.

SCREENING FOR PANCREATIC CANCER   Action Needed ◯

Routine screening for pancreatic cancer is not recommended, as the potential tests for this purpose (ultrasound, blood tests) are expensive and lack reliability.

SCREENING FOR BLADDER CANCER   Action Needed ◯

Blood in the urine is often the first sign of cancer of the bladder or of serious kidney disease. Blood in the urine may be present in such small amounts that it cannot be seen with the naked eye. In this situation, it can usually be detected by microscopic examination of the urine or by use of a chemically treated strip that is dipped into the urine. However, no major health organization, including the American Cancer Society, recommends screening for bladder cancer in asymptomatic adults.

SCREENING FOR ORAL CANCER   Action Needed ◯

The American Cancer Society recommends a cancer check-up that incorporates an oral exam every three years for people over age 20, and annually for those over age 40. The American Dental Association recommends having dental and oral check-ups twice a year. A complete oral examination should look for any signs of cancer or precancerous lesions. Regular examinations are especially important in people with risk factors predisposing them to oral cancer. This includes people who smoke or chew tobacco or who drink excessive amounts of alcohol, as well as people with suspicious sores in the mouth.

SCREENING FOR TUBERCULOSIS   Action Needed ○

The skin test for tuberculosis infection, the Mantoux skin test, should be performed on all people at increased risk of developing tuberculosis. These include:

- Household members of people with tuberculosis
- People in close contact with individuals with tuberculosis (e.g., medical personnel or nursing home staff members)
- Recent immigrants or refugees from countries where tuberculosis is common (e.g., Asia, Africa, Central and South America)
- Migrant workers
- Residents of nursing homes, correctional institutions and mental institutions
- Alcoholics
- IV drug users
- Medically underserved, low-income populations
- People with medical conditions that reduce resistance to tuberculosis (HIV infection, immune disorders)

SCREENING FOR RUBELLA (GERMAN MEASLES)   Action Needed ○

Rubella is a viral infection that generally causes a rash and swollen lymph nodes; this infection can result in serious problems if a woman is infected during pregnancy (severe complications may include miscarriage, stillbirth, as well as fetal growth retardation, hearing loss, and heart defects).

Blood testing for rubella antibodies should be performed on all pregnant and nonpregnant women of childbearing age (except those already known to be immune because of prior infection or immunization). Nonimmune, nonpregnant women (who agree not to become pregnant for three months) should be vaccinated. Nonimmune pregnant women should not be vaccinated until immediately after delivery.

Routine screening for rubella is not recommended for men.

SCREENING FOR HEPATITIS B   Action Needed ○

Hepatitis B is a viral infection affecting the liver that is most commonly transmitted through blood, contaminated needles and intimate contact. Additionally, it can be transmitted to a fetus while in utero or at the time of delivery if the mother is infected.

All pregnant women should be tested for hepatitis B at their first prenatal visit. Testing can be repeated in the third trimester for women engaged in high-risk behaviors such as:

- Intravenous drug use

- Suspected exposure to hepatitis B during pregnancy

Routine screening for hepatitis B is not recommended for men and nonpregnant women.

SCREENING FOR HIV INFECTION   Action Needed ◯

It is estimated that 800,000 to 1.2 million persons in the United States are infected with the human immunodeficiency virus (HIV, the virus that causes AIDS). A blood screening test for antibodies against HIV will reveal when an infection is present. However, after a person is infected, it can take weeks to months before he or she tests positive. Screening for HIV infection is recommended for anyone at increased risk for infection, including:

- Persons seeking treatment for sexually transmitted diseases

- Persons who have had multiple sexual partners

- Past or present intravenous drug users

- Homosexual and bisexual men

- Women or men whose past or present sexual partners were HIV-infected, had sex with men, or were intravenous drug users

- People with long-term residence or birth in an area with a high prevalence of HIV

- Prostitutes and their sex partners

- Individuals who received a blood transfusion between 1978 and 1985

Testing is also recommended for pregnant women (or women thinking about becoming pregnant) who are at high risk for HIV infection.

SCREENING FOR SYPHILIS   Action Needed ◯

Syphilis is a sexually transmitted disease caused by bacteria. If syphilis is left untreated, it can eventually cause very serious neurologic and cardiovascular complications. Routine blood testing for syphilis is recommended for both men and women with any of the following risk factors:

- Individuals with other sexually transmitted diseases (including HIV infection)

- People who engage in sex with multiple partners in geographic areas where syphilis is prevalent

- Sexual partners of people with active syphilis

- Prostitutes

In addition, all pregnant women should be tested at their first prenatal visit. Women at high risk of acquiring syphilis during their pregnancy (see risk factors noted above) should be retested during the third trimester and again at the time of delivery.

SCREENING FOR GONORRHEA   Action Needed ○

Gonorrhea is a sexually transmitted disease caused by bacteria. The screening test for a gonorrhea infection involves taking a specimen from the urethra in men or from the cervix in women for culture in the laboratory (the specimen is kept warm for a day or two and then examined under the microscope for evidence of bacterial growth). Routine cultures for gonorrhea should be obtained in the following high-risk groups of women:

- Young women (under age 25) with two or more sexual partners in the past year

- Women with a history of repeated bouts of gonorrhea

- Prostitutes

High-risk pregnant women should have gonorrhea cultures at their first prenatal visit. Repeat testing during the third trimester is recommended for women at risk of contracting gonorrhea during their pregnancy.

SCREENING FOR CHLAMYDIA   Action Needed ○

Chlamydia is the most common sexually transmitted disease caused by bacteria, with about three million new cases each year. Screening for a chlamydia infection is most commonly accomplished by culturing specimens taken from the cervix in women and the urethra in men. Blood and urine tests are also sometimes used for screening.

In 2001, the Task Force revised its guidelines for chlamydia screening, now recommending routine screening for:

- All sexually active women ages 25 years and younger.

- Other asymptomatic women at increased risk for infection (including those having more than one sexual partner, those having had a sexually transmitted disease in the past, and those not using condoms consistently and properly).

- All asymptomatic pregnant women ages 25 years and younger, as well as other pregnant women at increased risk for infection.

There are no recommendations for or against routine screening of asymptomatic women ages 26 and older at low risk for infection, as well as asymptomatic, low-risk pregnant women ages 26 and older. Routine screening for chlamydia is not recommended for men.

SCREENING FOR GENITAL HERPES SIMPLEX   Action Needed ○

Genital herpes is a sexually transmitted disease caused by a virus. Screening for this disease can be done through viral cultures taken from active sores or the genital area. This test is reliable when lesions are present, but much less so in the absence of active infection. Routine screening for genital herpes is not recommended for men and women without symptoms. However, the American College of Obstetricians and Gynecologists recommends that pregnant women be checked for active herpes lesions at the time of delivery; if test results are positive, a Cesarean section should be performed.

VISION SCREENING   Action Needed ○

Routine vision screening (with eye charts) of adolescents and nonelderly adults is not recommended by the Task Force, although periodic screening of the elderly is recommended. The American Academy of Ophthalmology, however, recommends regular eye exams for all adults after the age of 40.

SCREENING FOR GLAUCOMA   Action Needed ○

Glaucoma is a condition that causes the pressure within the eyeball to rise to abnormally high levels. It is the second leading cause of new cases of blindness in the United States. The screening test for glaucoma is called tonometry, which uses a device placed on the cornea or a puff of air blown against the cornea to measure the pressure inside the eye. The Task Force does not advocate routine testing for glaucoma, but for those at high risk of developing glaucoma, testing should be done periodically by an eye specialist. People at high risk include:

- Individuals with a family history of glaucoma

- Those with diabetes

- People of African-American descent over age 40, and Caucasians over age 65

- Individuals with severe myopia (or nearsightedness)

The American Academy of Ophthalmology recommends testing all adults periodically beginning at the age of 40.

SCREENING FOR HEARING IMPAIRMENT   Action Needed ○

Hearing screening tests are not recommended for adolescents and adults unless they are routinely exposed to loud noise. Elderly patients should have their hearing routinely evaluated and should be counseled about the availability and use of hearing aids.

SCREENING FOR CONGENITAL BIRTH DEFECTS

Several tests can be used during pregnancy to determine if abnormalities are present in the fetus. These include examination of the fetal genetic material, chromosome analysis, chemical tests for evidence of protein abnormalities associated with certain problems, and ultrasound examination to detect overt physical deformities.

Amniocentesis   Action Needed ○

Amniocentesis for chromosomal analysis should be offered to pregnant women age 35 and older. In younger women, amniocentesis is unnecessary unless there are special indications or circumstances.

Alpha-fetaprotein   Action Needed ○

Alpha-fetaprotein levels should be measured in pregnant women between weeks 16 and 18 of pregnancy. High levels of this protein in the blood of a pregnant women suggest the possibility of fetal abnormalities of the spinal cord or brain.

Ultrasound   Action Needed ○

Ultrasound examinations are not recommended as routine screening tests for birth defects.

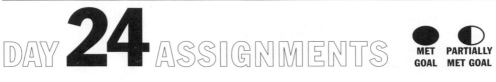

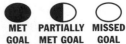

MET GOAL PARTIALLY MET GOAL MISSED GOAL

PHYSICAL VITALITY

1. Improve your time for the measured mile by 2 seconds.   **Time:**_____
2. Do all the flexibility and stretching exercises.
3. Do the leg and abdominal strength training exercises.

NUTRITIONAL VITALITY

4. Decrease total fat intake to 10% of total calories.
5. Eat at least 7 half-cup portions of fruits and vegetables.
6. Supplement as necessary to reach the vitamin & mineral recommendations.
7. Limit dietary cholesterol to 300 mg per day.
8. Limit sodium intake to 2,400 mg per day.
9. Consume at least 25 grams of dietary fiber per day.

MENTAL VITALITY

10. Spend at least 10 minutes practicing any deep relaxation technique.
11. Identify and eliminate as many sources of stress in your life as you can.
12. If you did not awaken this morning feeling rested, refreshed and looking forward to the day, make a commitment to increase the amount of time you sleep tonight by at least an hour.

EMOTIONAL & SPIRITUAL VITALITY

13. If you drink alcoholic beverages, limit your daily intake to one drink if you are a woman or 2 drinks if you are a man.
14. Answer this question: "If you learned that you had only one month to live, would you change the way you spent this day?"

MEDICAL VITALITY

15. Call your doctor to discuss any immunizations you might need based on the guidelines in this section.

ADULTS NEED IMMUNIZATIONS, TOO   DAY 24

Too many people think that immunizations are only for children. In fact, adults (and the elderly in particular) need immunizations, too. As is the case with children, adult immunizations save millions of dollars and much pain and suffering, and can even save lives.

As you get older, your immune system, your body's natural protection against infection, begins to "lose steam." As a result, you become more susceptible to infections. Immunizations boost your natural immunity and help your body fight off certain infectious illnesses. The U.S. Preventive Services Task Force makes the following recommendations for adults:

TETANUS-DIPHTHERIA TOXOID   Action Needed ○

Adults who have not received the primary series of the combined tetanus-diphtheria vaccine should be vaccinated. Also, all adults should be reimmunized (booster vaccine) at least once every ten years.

MEASLES   Action Needed ○

All persons born after 1956 who lack evidence of measles immunity (no record that they received the live vaccine on or after their first birthday, no laboratory evidence of immunity, and no history of measles infection) should be immunized. (Most people born prior to 1957 were exposed to the measles virus and developed immunity to the disease.) A second measles vaccine is advisable for teenagers and young adults in settings where many people congregate (such as high schools and colleges), if they have not previously received a second dose.

RUBELLA   Action Needed ○

Susceptible nonpregnant women of childbearing age (no proof of vaccination on or after their first birthday or laboratory evidence of immunity) who agree not to become pregnant for three months should be immunized. Susceptible pregnant women should be immunized following childbirth.

MUMPS   Action Needed ○

Susceptible men and women of any age should be immunized. This susceptible group includes individuals born after 1956 who lack laboratory evidence of immunity.

VARICELLA   Action Needed ○

The varicella zoster virus is responsible for the chickenpox and shingles. Healthy adults who have never had either a varicella infection or a previous varicella vaccination should receive two doses of the vaccine, administered four to eight weeks apart.

PNEUMOCOCCAL VACCINE   Action Needed ○

All men and women, 65 years of age and over, should be vaccinated at least once. The following groups of individuals under 65 years of age are considered to be at high risk for pneumococcal infection and should be immunized:

- People with certain medical conditions, including chronic heart or lung disease, diabetes, and persons who have had their spleen removed
- Institutionalized persons age 50 and over

- Anyone with immune deficiency may benefit from the vaccine, including alcoholics and people who have kidney or liver disease, sickle cell anemia, HIV infection, or certain cancers

INFLUENZA VACCINE   Action Needed ○

Individuals 65 years or older should be vaccinated annually (the best time for a flu shot is from mid-October to mid-November, just before the beginning of the flu season). Before the age of 65, the influenza vaccine should be administered to individuals who:

- Reside in chronic care facilities (e.g., nursing homes)
- Provide health care to a population at high risk for influenza (e.g., doctors, nurses)

- Have medical conditions such as heart or lung disease, diabetes, kidney disease, and immunosuppressive illnesses that put them at risk of infection

HEPATITIS A   Action Needed ○

Individuals at risk of exposure to hepatitis A require immunization, including:

- Persons traveling to or living in areas where the prevalence of hepatitis A is high, such as in Native American Pacific Islander and Alaska Native communities
- Military personnel

- Staff at day-care centers, and staff and patients at custodial institutions
- Hospital and laboratory workers
- Homosexual men
- Intravenous drug users

HEPATITIS B   Action Needed ○

All young adults not previously immunized should receive hepatitis B vaccine. Also, adults of any age deemed to be at high risk of infection require immunization, including:

- Homosexual men
- People traveling to countries where hepatitis B is prevalent
- IV drug users and their sexual partners
- Hemodialysis patients

- People with frequent occupational exposure to blood or blood products (e.g., doctors, nurses, laboratory personnel)
- People with multiple sexual partners in the previous six months

FOR ADDITIONAL INFORMATION

The Centers for Disease Control and Prevention can provide you with information on the vaccinations you may need when traveling to various countries. Call the CDC at (404) 332-4559.

ANTHRAX AND SMALLPOX: THREATS OF THE NEW CENTURY?

In the wake of the terrorist attacks of September 2001, words like "anthrax" and "smallpox" entered the vocabularies – and raised the anxiety levels – of millions of Americans. Because of the concern of biological warfare, many people have asked their doctors for information about anthrax and smallpox vaccines. Here's a brief review of these infectious diseases and the immunizations that have been developed against them.

Anthrax

Anthrax is an infection caused by a bacterium called *Bacillus anthracis*. It is found most commonly in animals such as cattle and sheep, but it can occur rarely in humans who are exposed to the bacteria. Most often, these bacteria enter the body through a cut or abrasion on the skin, but they can also be inhaled into the lungs or introduced into the gastrointestinal tract by the consumption of contaminated meat.

An anthrax immunization has been developed for use in humans. It consists of a series of three injections given at two-week intervals, followed by three additional injections administered 6, 12 and 18 months later. After that, annual booster shots are advised.

At present, the anthrax vaccine is recommended only for individuals considered at high-risk for exposure to the bacteria. This includes all active duty military personnel and people known to have been in contact with mail or other objects contaminated with the bacteria. Those with known exposures may also be offered a course of prophylactic antibiotic treatment.

At the time of this writing, there have been only about two dozen cases of cutaneous (skin) and inhalational anthrax in the U.S., and the Centers for Disease Control and Prevention considers the risk very low.

Smallpox

Smallpox is a highly infectious disease caused by the variola virus. As recently as the early 1950s, about 50 million cases occurred in the world each year, causing death in about 30 percent of cases. However, the availability of smallpox vaccine combined with a global eradication campaign completely eliminated the presence of smallpox worldwide by 1979. The following year, the World Health Organization advised that all countries cease using the vaccine.

Although effective, the smallpox vaccine has a risk of serious complications, so it is still not recommended except in individuals who face a genuine risk of exposure to the virus. When fears of bioterrorism emerged in late 2001, smallpox vaccine was in short supply, and government officials began stockpiling the vaccine for any future need. At the time of this writing, mass vaccination against smallpox was not recommended. (If you received the smallpox vaccination as a child, it may still provide some protection, although the degree of that protection may have diminished.)

DAY 25 ASSIGNMENTS

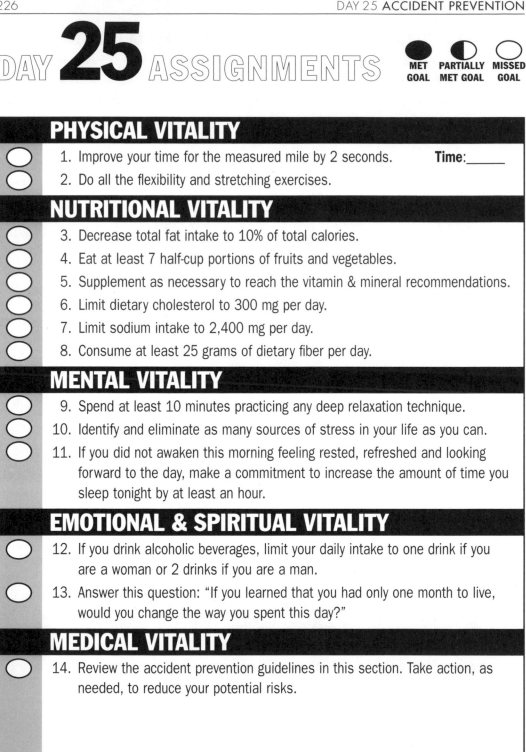

● MET GOAL   ◑ PARTIALLY MET GOAL   ○ MISSED GOAL

PHYSICAL VITALITY

1. Improve your time for the measured mile by 2 seconds.   **Time:**_____
2. Do all the flexibility and stretching exercises.

NUTRITIONAL VITALITY

3. Decrease total fat intake to 10% of total calories.
4. Eat at least 7 half-cup portions of fruits and vegetables.
5. Supplement as necessary to reach the vitamin & mineral recommendations.
6. Limit dietary cholesterol to 300 mg per day.
7. Limit sodium intake to 2,400 mg per day.
8. Consume at least 25 grams of dietary fiber per day.

MENTAL VITALITY

9. Spend at least 10 minutes practicing any deep relaxation technique.
10. Identify and eliminate as many sources of stress in your life as you can.
11. If you did not awaken this morning feeling rested, refreshed and looking forward to the day, make a commitment to increase the amount of time you sleep tonight by at least an hour.

EMOTIONAL & SPIRITUAL VITALITY

12. If you drink alcoholic beverages, limit your daily intake to one drink if you are a woman or 2 drinks if you are a man.
13. Answer this question: "If you learned that you had only one month to live, would you change the way you spent this day?"

MEDICAL VITALITY

14. Review the accident prevention guidelines in this section. Take action, as needed, to reduce your potential risks.

ACCIDENT PREVENTION   DAY 25

To ensure that you can maintain the *real* vitality you develop with our program, you need to actively practice accident prevention. Accidents at home, at work, or on the road kill thousands of people each year. In fact, recent government statistics show that only heart disease and cancer exceed accidents as leading causes of death in the United States. Here are some suggestions to reduce your risk of accidents:

NEVER DRINK AND DRIVE   Action Needed ○

More than half of all fatalities from car accidents involve alcohol and not all of them involve "drunk drivers." Just one cocktail puts you in danger by dulling your senses, slowing your reaction time and increasing your chances of falling asleep behind the wheel. And don't ever ride as a passenger in a car with a driver who's been drinking. It's as dangerous as driving under the influence of alcohol yourself.

ALWAYS WEAR YOUR SAFETY BELT   Action Needed ○

Several million people are injured each year in car accidents, and almost half of them require some form of medical treatment. Nearly 50,000 Americans die each year in motor vehicle accidents. Safety belts, if worn regularly by everyone, could reduce these numbers by half.

Wearing a safety belt not only protects your health, it spares your checkbook. A study by University of Chicago researchers compared injuries and hospital charges that safety belt and non-safety belt wearers incurred as a result of car accidents. People who wore safety belts suffered injuries that were significantly less severe and required admission to the hospital almost 65 percent less often.

Air bags also provide protection if you have an accident. But even if your car is equipped with air bags, that doesn't relieve you of the responsibility of buckling up. Your safety belt will hold you in position during an accident, allowing the air bag to do its job of protecting you. Also, because most air bags inflate only in head-on accidents, a buckled safety belt is necessary to keep you safe in any other type of car crash.

ALWAYS WEAR A BICYCLE HELMET   Action Needed ○

Each year there are more than a half-million emergency room visits and over 1,000 deaths resulting from biking accidents. Head injuries are the leading cause of death from these accidents. Yet, despite the fact that bicycle helmets have been shown to reduce the risk of head injury by as much as 85 percent, only 18 percent of bicyclists wear helmets always or sometimes. Be sure to wear a helmet every time you ride a bike.

INSTALL SMOKE DETECTORS AND FIRE ALARMS   Action Needed ○

If a fire occurs, the earlier you discover it, the greater your chance of putting it out or escaping from it. Today, your best tools for an early warning are smoke detectors; they can reduce your risk of dying in a fire by up to 67 percent.

Install smoke detectors throughout your home, mounting them on the ceiling or on the wall 6 to 12 inches from the ceiling. Place them in halls just outside bedrooms, and in the living room, garage and other areas where they can detect smoke as it approaches the bedrooms.

Remember that fire and smoke alarms are effective only if they're working. As many as one-third of installed alarms are thought to be inoperable, usually because their batteries are dead. You should check your alarms monthly to be sure they are working properly, and replace the batteries at least once a year.

Also, make sure that everyone in your household knows the escape routes out of your home in case of a fire. Keep a fire extinguisher in your house, too, placing it in or near the kitchen.

TURN DOWN YOUR WATER HEATER
TO 120 DEGREES FAHRENHEIT   Action Needed ○

A large number of scald burns occurs each year. This type of burn is excruciatingly painful and can cause permanent scarring and deformity.

Scald burns are most frequently caused by setting the hot water thermostat too high or by spilling hot cooking liquids on the skin. By turning down your central water heater, you can reduce the danger of an accidental burn in the tub or shower. It is important to lower your heater's temperature if you have a young child who is able to turn a bathtub faucet or an older person who could fall in the shower with the hot water running. Set your thermostat to no more than 120 degrees Fahrenheit. Anti-scald devices can be attached to faucets to automatically turn off the water if the temperature exceeds 120 degrees.

FOLLOW FIREARM SAFETY GUIDELINES   Action Needed ○

If you keep a firearm in your home for self-protection, you run the risk of a serious, often fatal accident. Studies show that for every case in which a gun is used successfully in shooting an intruder, there are 10 times as many instances of an injury caused by an accidental shooting, and a six-fold greater likelihood of an unintentional fatal shooting.

Removing firearms from your home is the best way to avoid an accidental shooting. But there are other steps you can take to reduce the risk associated with guns in your home. Studies show that almost one-third of firearm deaths could be prevented by using trigger locks and loading indicators, and by keeping guns unloaded and in a locked closet or cabinet. Anyone who keeps or uses guns should take firearm safety classes.

PREVENT FALLS   Action Needed ○

Accidental falls are a very common cause of injuries at any age, but the problem increases dramatically as people age and their muscles lose strength and their bones become more brittle. The loss of strength makes it much more difficult for them to "catch" themselves, while brittle bones increase the likelihood of fractures and other serious injuries.

Among older people living at home, about one-third will experience a fall in any given year. Among older people living in an institution, about two-thirds will have a fall in the same period of time. Of those who fall, about five percent will be seriously injured. Among people 65 or older, falls are responsible for about eight percent of all hospitalizations; they are the number-one cause for nursing home placement. In the elderly, the fractures caused by falls are a leading cause of severe disability and even death.

Nearly two-thirds of the falls at home could be prevented by removing physical hazards or making simple modifications to the environment. No matter what the age of the people in your household, go through the house and do the following:

- Attach all rugs and carpets securely to the floor at their edges so it is impossible to trip on a loose edge. If you use "throw" rugs, buy only those with a nonslip backing or nail the rugs to the floor.

- Eliminate all electrical cords and telephone cords that cross traffic paths.

- Install handrails in bathtubs, showers, and all other locations where a person may need some support.

- Put adhesive bath mats in tubs and showers.

- Make sure that all stepstools have handrails and rest solidly on their legs.

- Make sure all traffic areas, including stairways and hallways, are brightly lit.

Medications are another significant cause of falls, especially in the elderly. Many medications cause subtle changes in coordination and strength; others can make you dizzy or drowsy. Side effects can sometimes become overwhelming in the elderly, when slight changes in strength, coordination or gait can be enough to cause a fall. If you are having symptoms, review your medications and their potential side effects with your doctor. He or she may be able to switch you to another medication with fewer side effects, or lower the dose of the medication you are currently taking.

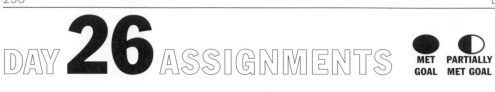

MET PARTIALLY MISSED
GOAL MET GOAL GOAL

PHYSICAL VITALITY

1. Improve your time for the measured mile by 2 seconds.   **Time**:_____
2. Do all the flexibility and stretching exercises.
3. Do the chest, back and arm strength training exercises.

NUTRITIONAL VITALITY

4. Decrease total fat intake to 10% of total calories.
5. Eat at least 7 half-cup portions of fruits and vegetables.
6. Supplement as necessary to reach the vitamin & mineral recommendations.
7. Limit dietary cholesterol to 300 mg per day.
8. Limit sodium intake to 2,400 mg per day.
9. Consume at least 25 grams of dietary fiber per day.

MENTAL VITALITY

10. Spend at least 10 minutes practicing any deep relaxation technique.
11. Identify and eliminate as many sources of stress in your life as you can.
12. If you did not awaken this morning feeling rested, refreshed and looking forward to the day, make a commitment to increase the amount of time you sleep tonight by at least an hour.

EMOTIONAL & SPIRITUAL VITALITY

13. If you drink alcoholic beverages, limit your daily intake to one drink if you are a woman or 2 drinks if you are a man.
14. Answer this question: "If you learned that you had only one month to live, would you change the way you spent this day?"

MEDICAL VITALITY

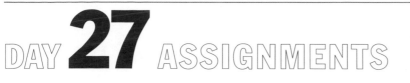 DAY **27** ASSIGNMENTS

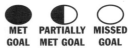
MET **PARTIALLY** **MISSED**
GOAL **MET GOAL** **GOAL**

PHYSICAL VITALITY

1. Improve your time for the measured mile by 2 seconds. **Time:**_____

2. Do all the flexibility and stretching exercises.

3. Do the leg and abdominal strength training exercises.

NUTRITIONAL VITALITY

4. Decrease total fat intake to 10% of total calories.

5. Eat at least 7 half-cup portions of fruits and vegetables.

6. Supplement as necessary to reach the vitamin & mineral recommendations.

7. Limit dietary cholesterol to 300 mg per day.

8. Limit sodium intake to 2,400 mg per day.

9. Consume at least 25 grams of dietary fiber per day.

MENTAL VITALITY

10. Spend at least 10 minutes practicing any deep relaxation technique.

11. Identify and eliminate as many sources of stress in your life as you can.

12. If you did not awaken this morning feeling rested, refreshed and looking forward to the day, make a commitment to increase the amount of time you sleep tonight by at least an hour.

EMOTIONAL & SPIRITUAL VITALITY

13. If you drink alcoholic beverages, limit your daily intake to one drink if you are a woman or 2 drinks if you are a man.

14. Answer this question: "If you learned that you had only one month to live, would you change the way you spent this day?"

MEDICAL VITALITY

VITALITY FOR LIFE   DAY 28

Four weeks ago, we promised that you could significantly increase your overall vitality level if you were willing to make small changes in your lifestyle and maintain them on a continuous basis. You made a promise, too – that you would follow this program as closely as you could for 28 days.

Now, you can determine if those promises paid off, by re-evaluating your health status and comparing it to where you were at the start of the program. Once you have done that, it's time to look toward the future, to determine how you will maintain and build upon the new level of vitality you have just achieved.

You can see how much progress you've made by completing the following questionnaire:

	FOUR WEEKS AGO	NOW
Weight:	_____	_____
Waist diameter:	_____	_____
Blood pressure:	_____	_____
Total cholesterol:	_____	_____
Time for mile:	_____	_____
Aerobic fitness	_____	_____
Flexibility	_____	_____
General strength	_____	_____
Vegetable, fruit portions/day	_____	_____
% fat in diet (est.)	_____	_____
Salt intake (high/low)	_____	_____
Adequate vitamin, mineral intake	_____	_____
Stress in control	_____	_____
Priorities right	_____	_____
Hours sleep/night	_____	_____
Anger level	_____	_____
No. drinks/day	_____	_____
OVERALL VITALITY LEVEL	_____	_____

WHAT'S NEXT

For the last 28 days, you've been able to rely on the structured program contained in this book to help you build vitality. Now, it's time for you to take over. Our program is ending, but yours is just beginning.

Your assignment today—after you complete the questionnaire on the opposite page— is to plan your own vitality program for the next 28 days and the rest of your life. Take time now to decide how you will structure your program, and how you will continue to record and monitor your progress.

Keep in mind that building a high level of vitality does not have to be complicated or difficult. It just requires small changes, applied consistently over time. Keep making those changes, and you can reach a level of vitality that you never dreamed possible.

If you are concerned about your ability to maintain a program all by yourself, you should give serious consideration to finding some outside support. Research shows that something as simple as getting a friend or relative to join you on your walks or joining an exercise group can make the difference between long-term adherence to a program and "dropping out." In the pages that follow, you'll find some helpful hints for getting professional support if you want it.

HOW TO CHOOSE A HEALTH CLUB

Are you thinking of joining a health club? How many times have you skipped a workout because the gym is too far away or will be too crowded when you get there? If you're like a lot of people, the answer is "too many."

Why give yourself an out? Cut the excuses by doing your homework and choosing a club that's right for you. It's no secret that picking a quality club is a key to sticking with your program. But choosing a health club can rank high on the confusion meter. Sign-up specials scream in all forms of the media, and it seems there's a new club on every corner. Before you jump on the latest two-for-one membership deal, take the time to consider these helpful tips from the American Council on Exercise (ACE):

- **Location.** For your fitness routine to be successful, exercise has to be convenient. You're more likely to use a club if it is close to either your home or workplace, although you don't want to choose a health club only because of its location. If you choose a club that isn't convenient, however, you are more likely to find an excuse to stop going. ACE offers referrals to clubs via its web site (www.acefitness.org).

- **Classes**. If classes are what keep you motivated, make sure the club offers an eclectic mix you like and that they are offered at a time of day that fits your schedule.

- **Staff**. Personal trainers and group fitness instructors should be certified through a nationally recognized certification organization like the American Council on

Exercise (ACE). Credible certification can assure you that the instructor meets the guidelines to provide a safe and efficient workout. ACE offers referrals to certified fitness professionals via its web site.

- **Hours**. Lots of health clubs open early and stay open late. Before you join, though, make sure your club is open when you plan to go. Then visit the club at the times you intend to work out. Check whether the club is too crowded or if there are long lines for equipment at that time.

- **Try It Before You Buy It.** Sales people are trained to hype the benefits of their health club, but you need to actually try out some of the equipment and get a feel for the club's atmosphere before you sign up. Request a day pass or a trial membership –this is a good way to "test drive" the health club's services.

- **Payments**. Many clubs have a variety of payment options. Find a payment schedule that meets your budget needs, and take advantage of any sign-up specials. Find out exactly what the membership fee is and what it includes. Will you have to pay extra for childcare and towels? Don't forget to ask if they require an initiation fee; and if you are joining a new club that hasn't opened yet, make sure that any deposits or payments are held in an escrow account until they officially open.

- **Reputation**. Before you join, talk to current members about their experiences with the club. The Better Business Bureau can tell you if the club is a member or if any complaints have been registered against it. Added security comes if the club is a member of the International Health, Racquet, and Sportsclub Association (IHRSA). IHRSA clubs must adhere to a code of ethics that protects the health and safety of their members, as well as protects consumers from unscrupulous business practices. To find an IHRSA club in your area, go to www.healthclubs.com or call (800) 766-1278.

- **Little Details.** As you tour the club, pay attention to details. How clean is the facility? Is the music too loud? Is most of the equipment in working order? Too many "out of order" signs may indicate poor maintenance. Are new members provided with a club orientation and instruction on how to use the equipment? Make sure the club is a place where you would enjoy spending time.

With a little research and patience, you will be rewarded with a membership at a health club you can call "home." More importantly, you will be reaping the long-term benefits of a structured exercise program that perfectly suits your lifestyle.

©American Council on Exercise (ACE); reprinted with permission

HOW TO CHOOSE A PERSONAL TRAINER

A personal trainer can help keep you motivated in your exercise program, and make sure you're doing your workouts properly. Here are some recommendations from the American Council on Exercise for selecting a trainer.

A personal trainer should be certified. This certification is your assurance that the trainer has the knowledge to provide you with a safe and effective workout. But not just any certification will do. You want a personal trainer who has been certified by a nationally recognized certifying organization, like ACE, which is the largest non-profit fitness-certifying organization in the world.

Certification is more than a piece of paper. For example, to qualify for ACE certification, a personal trainer has to pass an intensive three-and-a-half hour, 175-question exam that covers exercise science and programming knowledge, including anatomy, kinesiology, health screening, basic nutrition, and instructional methods.

After checking certification, there are a few other factors you should take into consideration when hiring a personal trainer. Many require asking direct questions.

A Checklist to Help You Hire The Right Personal Trainer:

- **Ask for references.** Ask the trainer for the names and phone numbers of other clients with goals similar to yours. Call to see if they were pleased with their workouts, if the trainer was punctual and prepared, and if they felt their individual needs were addressed. The best personal trainers are those given high marks by others.
- **Make sure the trainer has liability insurance and provides business policies in writing.** Many personal trainers operate as independent contractors and are not employees of a fitness facility. You should find out if the trainer you want to hire carries professional liability insurance. A reputable personal trainer should also make sure you understand the cancellation policy and billing procedure. The best way to avoid confusion and to protect your rights is to have those policies in writing.
- **Look for a personal trainer who is able to assist you with your special needs.** A personal trainer should always have you fill out a health history questionnaire to determine your needs or limitations. If you have a medical condition or a past injury, a personal trainer should design a session that takes these into account. If you're under a doctor's care, a personal trainer should discuss any exercise concerns with your doctor, and should ask for a health screening or release from your doctor.
- **Find out what the trainer charges.** Rates vary, depending on the trainer's experience and the length and location of the workout session. For example, a personal trainer who works in a fitness club will probably charge less per hour than one who works independently and needs to come to your home or office.

- **Decide if this is someone you can work with.** Some people like to exercise in the morning, some in the evening. Will the personal trainer you're talking to accommodate your schedule? What about the trainer's gender? Some people do better working with a trainer of the same sex; others prefer the opposite sex.

The personal trainer you select should motivate you by positive, not negative, reinforcement. Even more important, that trainer should be someone you like.

Ask yourself if you think you could get along well with the trainer. Ask yourself, too, if you think the trainer is genuinely interested in helping you.

The personal trainer who best measures up is the one to hire. He or she is the professional who will help you get the best results.

©American Council on Exercise (ACE); reprinted with permission

HOW TO CHOOSE AN ONLINE PERSONAL TRAINER

Today, many personal trainers are riding the dot-com wave, making their services more accessible and affordable than ever. Despite the obvious benefits of online training, cyber-training is most effective as a supplement to working one-on-one with a qualified trainer. (Due to the complexity of many strength-training and conditioning programs, novice exercisers should begin with a hands-on trainer.)

On average, hands-on personal trainers charge between $35 and $100 per hour, depending on the market, while their cyber counterparts are available at a fraction of the cost, with some charging as little as $10 per month. Online training is also accessible to anyone with a computer and modem, making it possible for busy travelers or people in remote areas to have access to a personal trainer. This type of training is recommended primarily for intermediate and advanced exercisers or those with very specific goals such as training for a marathon or triathlon.

Consider the following tips for picking and utilizing a safe and effective online personal trainer.

- First and foremost, check the qualifications of the staff who will be training you. Sites should provide background information about their staff. Make sure the personal trainers have a college degree in an exercise-related field and/or are certified by a well-known organization such as the American Council on Exercise (ACE), the American College of Sports Medicine (ACSM), or the National Strength and Conditioning Association (NSCA). To check if a trainer is certified by ACE, call 800-825-3636. If the site offers nutritional advice, make sure registered dietitians are on staff.

- Inquire about the trainers' experience with your age group or with your particular needs or health challenges (e.g., specialization with older adults, weight management). Be wary of sites that rely on "celebrity trainers" or professional athletes to sell their services; it's important to find out who will actually be designing your workouts. And always avoid sites that make exaggerated claims or guarantee fitness results.

- Make sure the site is easy to navigate. If it's too complicated you probably won't stick with it. Some companies will allow you to "tour" the site before signing up.

- Look for a sample workout plan. If available, make sure the plans are thorough and detailed (e.g., weight, sets, repetitions, intensity) and not simply a list of exercises. Also determine whether the site provides a method for visually communicating proper exercise technique; text-only instructions can be difficult to follow.

- The site should provide an easy means of contacting your trainer for questions or concerns. Most sites provide e-mail contact, but also look for sites that have a toll-free number so you can actually speak to a trainer. Questions should be addressed in a timely manner.

- Look for a site that provides bulletin board-type forums and online group support that you can use to communicate with other exercisers with similar goals.

- Finally, avoid training sites that "prescribe" nutritional supplement programs. Trainers should not be advising you on nutrition (beyond the food guide pyramid) unless they are registered dietitians.

- Once you've decided to sign up, make sure the site requires you to complete a detailed health-history questionnaire. This evaluation should address, among other things, your goals, present level of fitness, and health concerns. Trainers need this information to customize a program to fit your needs. Online exercisers should be honest when filling out the evaluation forms; in other words, don't lie about your age, weight or experience level as this could reduce the effectiveness of your training program and possibly lead to injury.

- Determine whether the workouts are truly customized for you. Some sites use computer programs to provide preset workout plans based on how you answer their evaluation form. If you receive a plan immediately, a computer likely created your workout. These plans are fine for some exercisers, but you may wish to find a site that provides you with a more personalized fitness program.

- Is your program updated regularly? Does the site have online exercise logs and do you receive e-mail responses or postings that address your progress?

If you are unhappy with the answers to these questions, or with the service of the site you have chosen, don't hesitate to request a refund and seek another more suitable online personal trainer. To experience the benefits of a personal trainer, virtual or otherwise, you must feel completely comfortable and confident in his or her ability to help you reach your health and fitness goals.

©*American Council on Exercise (ACE); reprinted with permission*

APPENDIX: VITAMINS

VITAMIN A

Vitamin A is not just a single nutrient, but a group of compounds that are structurally related and act in similar biological ways. The group includes two general categories: retinoids (preformed vitamin A) and carotenoids (precursors of vitamin A). Carotenoids, the pigments that give plant life its red, orange, and yellow hues, are plentiful in many common fruits and vegetables, from sweet potatoes to apricots, from cantaloupes to carrots. Large amounts of beta carotene—the best-known carotenoid, and the most abundant and most important nutritionally—are found in yellow and orange fruits and vegetables in particular. In contrast to retinoids, carotenoids exist only in plants.

Whether you consume vitamin A in its preformed state or your body manufactures it from precursors, your liver stores it and your body uses it as needed; therefore, you do not necessarily need to consume this vitamin every day. Whenever taking preformed vitamin A, you should be aware that excessive amounts of it can accumulate in your body and lead to troublesome—even dangerous—toxic side effects.

To meet your body's vitamin A requirements, you can consume either preformed retinoids or carotenoids such as beta carotene. Like vitamin A itself, beta carotene is fat-soluble. It has some distinct advantages over vitamin A, however, especially with respect to toxicity. For one thing, beta carotene itself is nontoxic. For another, the body can decrease conversion of beta carotene to vitamin A when blood levels of vitamin A are high. When you increase your intake of vitamin A and beta carotene, the body's conversion process automatically slows down.

Health Benefits

The body of evidence supporting the health benefits of vitamin A and beta carotene is growing rapidly. For example:

Cancer. A number of studies have shown persuasively that beta carotene and vitamin A have a protective effect against lung cancer. Although two studies have suggested that beta carotene could *increase* the risk of lung cancer in smokers, the majority of about 200 published reports have shown that the nutrient offers positive benefits. Other types of cancer—including stomach cancer and breast cancer—have occurred less often when intakes and blood levels of vitamin A or beta carotene were high, although not every study has produced such positive results.

Cardiovascular Disease. The findings of several major studies suggest that beta carotene may help decrease the risk of cardiovascular disease. However, some studies have shown no protective benefits, and experts must await the results of ongoing studies before drawing any conclusions.

HIV Infection. Vitamin A and beta carotene may offer hope for individuals whose immune system function is impaired, particularly people with acquired immune deficiency syndrome, or AIDS. A study at Johns Hopkins University, which compared vitamin A levels in people who tested positive versus those testing negative for the virus causing AIDS, concluded that the vitamin is necessary for normal functioning of the immune system, and that a deficiency "seems to be an important risk factor for disease progression" in the serious viral infection.

Eye Disorders. Researchers have found that beta carotene has a protective effect against common eye disorders such as cataracts and macular degeneration. For instance, in a study at Tufts University and other Boston-area institutions, the risk of developing cataracts was significantly higher in individuals with low blood levels of beta carotene. These findings have been supported by research at the University of Tampere in Finland and other medical centers

Who's At Risk For Vitamin A Deficiency?

If you answer yes to any of the following questions, you (or your child) have an above-average risk of developing a vitamin A deficiency.

- *Do you have chronic diarrhea, chronic pancreatitis, cystic fibrosis, or chronic liver disease (including hepatitis, cirrhosis, or liver cancer)?* Chronic diarrhea reduces the absorption of vitamin A. Liver diseases can reduce the amount of vitamin A stored by the body.

- *Do you consume large amounts of alcohol?* Alcohol reduces the levels of vitamin A and/or beta carotene in the liver.

- *Do you smoke cigarettes?* Cigarette smoking decreases the level of beta carotene in the blood.

- *Do you regularly take any medications that can interfere with your body's absorption of vitamin A from the intestinal tract?* Such medications include certain drugs within the following categories: (1) cholesterol-lowering medications (colestipol and cholestyramine); (2) mineral oil (which attaches itself to vitamin A and carries it out through the intestinal tract); and (3) birth-control pills (which increase levels of retinol in the bloodstream and decrease liver stores of the vitamin, which may increase the body's vitamin A needs).

- *Are you under a lot of stress?* Stress can reduce the level of retinol in the blood, probably by increasing the number of free radicals present and possibly by causing the body to break down vitamin A more quickly. Stress caused by overwork, fatigue, a fever, a chronic infection, or even too much exercise can have this effect on vitamin A levels.

- *Are you pregnant or breast-feeding?* If so, your body needs more vitamin A than usual.

- *Does your child avoid foods that are good sources of vitamin A?* Because of their rapid growth and faster metabolism, youngsters probably require more vitamin A, on a pound-for-pound basis, than adults.

The Consequences of a Vitamin A Deficiency

Vitamin A can be stored in the liver and released into the bloodstream for use by the body as needed, so we don't need to consume vitamin A every day to prevent signs of deficiency. For that reason, *occasional* dietary deficiencies will probably not cause major deficiency symptoms. However, chronic vitamin A deficiency can cause obvious deficiency symptoms, some of them serious.

Night blindness, for example, is an early symptom of vitamin A deficiency, although it is reversible. But chronic deficiency can lead to a more serious condition—a drying of the eyes called *xerosis*—which may cause ulcerations of the cornea. A deficiency of this nutrient can increase the body's vulnerability to certain types of infections, particularly in the respiratory tract (sore throats, sinus infections). Vitamin A deficiency can also interfere with normal growth in children by impairing bone growth.

Other deficiency-related conditions include *follicular hyperkeratosis*, in which the skin assumes a rough texture and the senses of smell and taste may be lost. Deficiencies can also affect reproduction, including a decreased ability of the body to manufacture sperm, spontaneous abortion (miscarriage), abnormal menstruation, or birth defects.

What Are the Best Food Sources?

Many common foods are rich in vitamin A. This important nutrient occurs naturally only in foods of animal origin, such as dairy products (milk, cheese, butter, and ice cream), egg yolks, fish (and fish oils), and liver and other internal organs. Other food products have been fortified with vitamin A, including margarine, breakfast cereals, and milk.

We obtain much of our vitamin A indirectly from the carotenoids, including beta carotene, found in many vegetables and fruits—for instance, yellow and orange vegetables (carrots, sweet potatoes, and pumpkins), green leafy vegetables (spinach, broccoli, collard greens, turnip greens, and peppers), and yellow and orange fruits (papayas, oranges, apricots, peaches, and cantaloupes).

While nutrient tables are useful guides for vitamin A and beta carotene intake, they are not always helpful for precise assessments. The amount of vitamin A in a product can vary, particularly in meat and dairy products, depending on the diet of the animal that the product came from. The content of carotenoids can vary, too, depending on growing conditions for the fruits and vegetables. The processing and storage of foods can also alter these values: Both vitamin A and beta carotene are insoluble in water, they are relatively unstable in heat, and exposure to light can destroy both of these nutrients.

DR. ART ULENE'S RECOMMENDATION FOR VITAMIN A AND MIXED CAROTENOIDS

My recommendation for the daily intake of vitamin A is 5,000 IU, which equals the USRDA for adults. No toxic side effects have been reported at this dosage. I recommend 6 to 15 mg of beta carotene per day (formal RDAs have not been established for this nutrient). But total quantity is only part of my recommendation. To avoid toxicity altogether, I believe everyone should obtain a significant portion of their vitamin A by consuming mixed carotenoids. By using carotenoids to help reach your vitamin A goal, you sidestep the risk of toxicity and, at the same time, get some additional antioxidant benefits from the carotenoids themselves.

I recommend that you consume 6 to 15 mg of beta carotene or mixed carotenoids per day. Note that 15 mg is equivalent to about 25,000 IU of vitamin A, but in this form it is perfectly safe.

It is possible to consume 5,000 IU (or 1,000 mcg) of vitamin A and 6 to 15 mg of beta carotene or mixed carotenoids each day solely through diet. Most people don't, however, and could benefit from supplementation. According to the government's Continuing Survey of Food Intakes by Individuals, women consumed an average of 953 mcg of vitamin A per day in the mid-1990s, which is a little below my recommendation. However, the average woman consumed only 0.5 mg of carotenes per day, far below by recommendation of 6 to 15 mg.

VITAMIN B₃—NIACIN

The name niacin is commonly applied to two natural, active compounds: nicotinic acid and nicotinamide (also called niacinamide). If you feel uneasy about the similarity of those names to nicotine, the addictive substance in tobacco, you need not worry. In fact, these compounds are not chemically related to the dangerous soundalike. Because researchers feared that the public might confuse them, however, the more generic term niacin was used to represent both nicotinic acid and nicotinamide. Niacin is now accepted as the name for vitamin B_3.

In concert with a variety of enzymes, niacin participates in a variety of metabolic processes. It helps convert energy derived from carbohydrates, fats, and protein into a form that the body can use.

Health Benefits

In large doses, niacin (specifically, nicotinic acid) positively affects fats in the blood. It can decrease total cholesterol, while increasing the HDL ("good") component of cholesterol. One of the best known studies of niacin's effects on cholesterol is the Coronary Drug Project, which found that a group of men with coronary heart disease experienced a lower average cholesterol level when taking niacin (3 grams a day), compared to those taking a cholesterol-lowering medication (clofibrate) or placebo. Equally impressive was the finding that men taking niacin had fewer life-threatening coronary events such as heart attacks.

Who's At Risk For Niacin Deficiency?

If you answer yes to any of the following questions, you have an above-average risk of developing a niacin deficiency.

- *Do you exercise?* The more energy you expend, the more niacin you need, because niacin plays a role in converting foods into energy.

- *Are you pregnant?* Because pregnant women require more energy, they need more niacin. The RDAs advise an additional 2 mg per day during pregnancy.

- *Are you breast-feeding?* Women who are nursing lose niacin in their breast milk and also expend more energy; thus they need extra niacin.

The Consequences of a Niacin Deficiency

The symptoms seen most frequently among individuals who are niacin-deficient are skin disorders. The skin becomes dry, cracked, and scaly, and may appear to be darkly pigmented, particularly in areas exposed to sunlight, including the forehead, neck, and backs of the hands. Niacin deficiency also affects the nervous system, leading to irritability, anxiety, depression, tremors, muscle weakness, confusion, and disorientation.

What Are the Best Food Sources?

Meats and nuts are good sources of niacin. So are poultry, fish, and whole-grain and enriched breads. Many cereals are also enriched with niacin.

Keep in mind that the amino acid tryptophan, after going through a conversion process in the body, also provides us with niacin. Milk, eggs, and corn have limited amounts of niacin in them but are good sources of tryptophan, and are therefore wise choices for maintaining a high niacin level.

Niacin is a stable vitamin and withstands high temperatures and exposure to oxygen. Because it dissolves in water, though, cooking in liquid will partially leach niacin content from food.

DR. ART ULENE'S RECOMMENDATION FOR NIACIN

To meet the needs of most active adults, my recommendation for niacin is 20 mg (niacin equivalents) per day, which is equal to the USRDA for adults. No toxic side effects have been reported at this dosage.

According to government statistics, about 67 percent of adult women and 80 percent of adult men consume the RDA of niacin through diet alone, and thus many people fall short of the recommendations. Thus, you may find it necessary to take a niacin supplement each day.

VITAMIN B_6—PYRIDOXINE

Scientists first firmly identified and described vitamin B_6 and its structure in 1939. Today, we know that this vitamin exists naturally in foods in three closely related forms: pyridoxine, pyridoxal, and pyridoxamine. Nutrition supplements generally provide B_6 in the form of pyridoxine.

Health Benefits

Studies have shown that vitamin B_6 may be useful in the prevention of coronary heart disease because it helps reduce blood levels of the amino acid homocysteine. High levels of homocysteine in the blood have been associated with damage to the artery walls and atherosclerosis. Because of this link between elevated homocysteine levels and coronary heart disease, many doctors now recommend supplementation with vitamin B_6.

Who's At Risk For Vitamin B_6 Deficiency?

If you answer yes to any of the following questions, you have an above-average risk of developing a vitamin B_6 deficiency.

- *Are you pregnant?* Women who are pregnant or have just given birth require extra vitamin B_6. The RDA suggests an additional 0.6 mg of B_6 during pregnancy.
- *Are you breast-feeding?* Women who breast-feed can lose as much as 0.25 mg of vitamin B_6 per liter of milk. The RDAs advise an additional 0.5 mg of B_6 per day when breast-feeding.

- *Are you taking certain drugs, such as isoniazid (to treat tuberculosis), hydralazine (for high blood pressure), or penicillamine (for rheumatoid arthritis)?* These drugs can increase the body's excretion of vitamin B_6 in the urine.

- *Are you taking birth-control pills?* Blood levels of vitamin B_6 decrease 15 to 20 percent in women taking birth-control pills. The reasons for this are not clear.

- *Does your diet include a lot of protein?* Vitamin B_6 plays an important role in protein metabolism, so the more protein you consume, the more vitamin B_6 you need.

- *Do you drink a lot of alcohol?* Some 20 to 30 percent of alcoholics experience a vitamin B_6 deficiency.

The Consequences of a Vitamin B_6 Deficiency

Although rare, vitamin B_6 deficiencies can produce skin disorders, such as scaling of the skin. Inflammation of the tongue and mucous membranes of the mouth may also occur. Other symptoms include depression, irritability, dizziness, and weakness, as well as convulsions, which more frequently occur in infants. Additional symptoms include anemia, weakened immune function, and nausea and vomiting.

What Are the Best Food Sources?

Many common foods are rich in vitamin B_6. If your diet includes liver, fish, pork, soybeans, wheat germ, peanuts, or walnuts, for example, you are getting B_6 in your meals. Dairy products, most vegetables, and fruits (with the exception of bananas) contain relatively little B_6.

When preparing foods, remember that vitamin B_6 is water-soluble, and significant amounts of vitamin B_6 can be lost in processing and cooking.

DR. ART ULENE'S RECOMMENDATION FOR VITAMIN B_6

My recommendation for the daily intake of vitamin B_6 is 4 mg per day, which is double the USRDA of 2 mg per day. My recommended dosage will help to reduce blood levels of homocysteine, which in turn can reduce the risk of coronary heart disease. This dosage will also compensate for the additional needs of women who use oral contraceptives and people who consume large amounts of protein or alcohol. No toxic side effects have been reported at this dosage.

While you could consume enough vitamin B_6 in your diet alone, only about 37 percent of women and 47 percent of men consume even the RDA for this vitamin, according to recent government statistics. Thus, to reach my recommended dose of 4 mg, you may need to take a daily supplement.

VITAMIN B₁₂—COBALAMIN

The history of vitamin B_{12} dates back to the 19th century, when a ferocious form of anemia swept through parts of Europe. This disease was so fierce that it was often called pernicious anemia. No one was sure what caused it or how to treat it, but years later, it was finally determined that foods rich in B_{12} could combat it. Today, because the B_{12} molecule contains the trace element cobalt, some supplement labels list this vitamin as cobalamin. Like other B vitamins, vitamin B_{12} is water-soluble.

In order for your body to absorb the vitamin B_{12} that you consume, cells in the stomach lining must produce a protein called intrinsic factor. Without enough of this factor in the gastric juices, the intestines cannot absorb B_{12}, and a deficiency may occur.

Health Benefits

Vitamin B_{12} plays a part in preventing cardiovascular disease by helping to reduce blood levels of the amino acid homocysteine. High homocysteine levels have been associated with the buildup of plaque along the inside walls of the arteries, increasing the risk of angina, heart attack, and stroke. Recently, scientists have discovered that vitamin B_{12}, vitamin B_6, and folic acid are all important factors in the breakdown of homocysteine in the body, keeping the amino acid from building up to toxic levels and accumulating in the arteries. Supplementation with these B vitamins may help normalize homocysteine levels, thereby reducing the risk of cardiovascular disease.

Who's At Risk For Vitamin B₁₂ Deficiency?

If you answer yes to any of the following questions, you have an above-average risk of developing a vitamin B_{12} deficiency.

- *Are you a strict vegetarian?* Vitamin B_{12} exists naturally only in animal foods and products. Children on vegetarian diets are particularly susceptible to deficiencies, because they have not yet built up stores of B_{12} in their liver.
- *Are you an older person?* Older people often have more trouble absorbing B_{12} than younger people do, because their bodies have more difficulty producing the intrinsic factor that enables them to absorb B_{12}.
- *Do you have tapeworms?* Although rare, tapeworms can cause a vitamin B_{12} deficiency.
- *Are you taking medications such as colchicine (for gout), cholestyramine (for high cholesterol levels), or omeprazole (for ulcers)?* These medications interfere with the absorption of vitamin B_{12}. Particular antibiotics, such as neomycin, can lower B_{12} levels, although scientists do not yet understand why.

- *Have parts of your stomach been surgically removed?* Intrinsic factor, which is important for absorption of B_{12}, is produced in the stomach.
- *Are you pregnant?* A fetus needs 0.1 to 0.2 mcg of vitamin B_{12} per day. According to the RDAs, pregnant women should consume an additional 0.2 mcg of vitamin B_{12} daily.
- *Are you breast-feeding?* A baby gets about 0.6 mcg of vitamin B_{12} per liter of breast milk. According to the RDAs, breast-feeding women should take an extra 0.6 mcg of B_{12} per day.

The Consequences of a Vitamin B_{12} Deficiency

Vitamin B_{12} deficiency is most commonly associated with pernicious anemia, a condition that is characterized by weakness and fatigue, weight loss, diarrhea, sore tongue, and pale skin. Severe deficiency can cause impaired nervous system function and even permanent nerve damage. Psychological disturbances, including moodiness and depression, are also warning signs of vitamin B_{12} deficiency.

What Are the Best Food Sources?

Foods of animal origin are excellent—and the only natural—sources of vitamin B_{12}. Meats (including liver and kidney), fish, poultry, milk, and cheese all contain this vitamin.

If you are a vegetarian, vitamin B_{12} supplements are probably a good choice. Soybean milk substitutes and breakfast cereals are often vitamin B_{12}-fortified.

The vitamin is water-soluble but is very stable in the presence of heat, so little vitamin B_{12} is lost in cooking.

DR. ART ULENE'S RECOMMENDATION FOR VITAMIN B_{12}

Until recently, I recommended 5 mcg of vitamin B_{12} per day. However, because of the important role that vitamin B_{12} plays in controlling levels of homocysteine, I have greatly raised my recommended level—to 100 mcg per day. This is many times higher than the USRDA (which is 6 mcg per day), but I feel justified because high homocysteine levels probably increase the risk of coronary heart disease very significantly. There are no toxic side effects associated with this level of vitamin B_{12} intake.

The average man in the U.S. consumes nearly 8 mcg of vitamin B_{12} per day; the average intake for women is close to 5 mcg. In both cases, the consumption of B_{12} is well above the USRDA but far below my recommendation. In fact, you'd have great difficulty meeting our recommended level through diet alone unless you were eating many pounds of fish, or entire boxes of fortified breakfast cereal every day.

VITAMIN B₁—THIAMIN

Thiamin or vitamin B_1, the first of the B vitamins to be discovered, was initially isolated in the mid-1920s. Along with the other vitamins in the B-complex family, thiamin facilitates the work of every cell in the body.

Health Benefits

Today we know that thiamin plays an important part in changing energy stored in carbohydrates to a form that our bodies can use. Thiamin is also necessary for the nervous system to function properly, and it may be involved with producing chemical messengers in the brain called neurotransmitters.

Who's At Risk For Thiamin Deficiency?

If you answer yes to any of the following questions, you have an above-average risk of developing a thiamin deficiency.

- *Do you have diabetes?* This condition can increase the amount of thiamin excreted in the urine.

- *Do you have a disorder that increases your metabolic rate?* Such disorders, including infections, fevers, hyperactivity, and hyperthyroidism, increase thiamin requirements.

- *Do you consume large amounts of alcohol?* Alcohol interferes with the absorption of thiamin, and alcoholics tend to have poor diets that may be deficient in thiamin.

- *Do you eat large amounts of raw fish?* An enzyme called thiaminase, found in raw fish, inactivates thiamin; cooking, however, destroys this enzyme.

- *Do you consume large amounts of carbohydrates?* Your body needs thiamin to metabolize carbohydrates. The more carbohydrates you consume, therefore, the more thiamin you require.

- *Are you pregnant or breast-feeding?* According to the RDAs, women should take an additional .4 mg of thiamin per day during pregnancy to accommodate for their own increased needs and for the growth of the fetus. Women who are breast-feeding should take an additional .5 mg of thiamin per day to compensate for the amount of the vitamin lost in breast milk.

The Consequences of a Thiamin Deficiency

Severe thiamin deficiency can result in the development of *beriberi*, a disease that causes a number of diverse symptoms. Beriberi's effects on the nervous system can include loss of muscle strength, leg spasms, and leg muscle paralysis. Psychological disturbances, such as mental confusion and depression, may also be brought about by this deficiency disease.

People who live in developed countries are relatively safe from vitamin B₁ deficiency and beriberi, due to the wide availability of a variety of foods that contain the vitamin. However, people who abuse alcohol are most likely to develop deficiency symptoms, not only because alcohol interferes with the body's absorption of thiamin, but it also may crowd foods with adequate nutrients out of the diet.

What Are the Best Food Sources?

Thiamin is present in many foods. Some of the best sources include whole-grain or enriched breads and cereals, brewer's yeast, liver and other organ meats, lean cuts of pork, peas, beans, and nuts and seeds.

Heat or immersion of foods in water during cooking can destroy thiamin. To retain this water-soluble vitamin, cook thiamin-containing foods in only small amounts of water.

DR. ART ULENE'S RECOMMENDATION FOR THIAMIN

I recommend a range of 1.5 to 10 mg of thiamin per day. That compares to a USRDA of 1.5 mg per day. This low level (1.5 mg) is acceptable for many people, but higher levels are more appropriate for anyone who is extremely active, and for those who consume large amounts of carbohydrates, because thiamin plays an important role in the metabolism of carbohydrates for energy. Higher levels of thiamin consumption are also important for men and women who already have liver disease or who have an increased risk of liver disease because of excessive alcohol consumption.

Surveys taken in the mid-1990s found that only about 63 percent of women and 69 percent of men consume the RDA of thiamin in their diets.

VITAMIN B₂—RIBOFLAVIN

Toward the end of the 19th century, a fluorescent pigment was detected in milk whey; subsequently, the pigment was found in other sources (liver and eggs) as well. Although its significance was not initially understood, we have come to appreciate its growth-promoting properties. In the 1930s, the nutrient was isolated and identified. It was vitamin B₂, or riboflavin.

Health Benefits

Like other B vitamins, riboflavin is important to the complex processes in your body that give you energy from the foods you consume. Riboflavin is part of two coenzymes involved in the metabolism of carbohydrates, fats and proteins. This vitamin is also essential for the normal growth and repair of all body tissues.

Who's At Risk For Riboflavin Deficiency?

If you answer yes to any of the following questions, you have an above-average risk of developing a riboflavin deficiency.

- *Do you chronically take medications such as diuretics, phobenicid (an anti-gout drug), or antidepressants (tricyclics)?* Diuretics and phobenicid increase the excretion of riboflavin in the urine; antidepressants interfere with the metabolism of riboflavin.

- *Do you have diabetes?* Diabetics tend to excrete increased amounts of riboflavin in their urine.

- *Do you exercise, even moderately?* As you expend energy, you use riboflavin more rapidly.

- *Are you pregnant or breast-feeding?* The RDAs advise taking an additional .3 mg of riboflavin per day during pregnancy, an additional .5 mg per day during the first six months of breast-feeding, and an additional .4 mg for longer periods of breast-feeding.

The Consequences of a Riboflavin Deficiency

Initial signs of a riboflavin deficiency tend to be general in nature, including loss of appetite and reduced growth. This is followed by the appearance of localized deficiency symptoms, such as sores, cracks, and dry or scaly skin on the nose, lips, and corners of the mouth; inflamed tongue and loss of the sense of taste; eye disorders, such as tearing, burning, reddened eyes and a decrease in the sharpness of vision; and anemia. Changes in behavior—including depression, nervousness, and irritability—may also result from damage to the nervous system.

What Are the Best Food Sources?

Generous amounts of riboflavin are available in milk and other dairy foods, including cheese, ice cream, and yogurt. (The higher the fat content of a dairy food, the less riboflavin it has.) Meats (especially liver and other organ meats) and fish (including salmon and tuna) are also good sources of riboflavin, as are enriched grain products and green leafy vegetables such as broccoli and spinach.

Exposure to sunlight and ultraviolet light can destroy riboflavin. It is important, therefore, to store riboflavin-rich foods in refrigerators, cupboards, and opaque containers that guard them from sunlight.

DR. ART ULENE'S RECOMMENDATION FOR RIBOFLAVIN

My recommendation for the daily intake of riboflavin is 2 to 5 mg per day, which is higher than the USRDA (1.7 mg). This recommended dosage will also compensate for the additional needs of people who have diabetes or use diuretics or tricyclic antidepressant medications. No toxic side effects have been reported at this dosage.

Recent government surveys show that only 61 percent of adult women and 71 percent of adult men consume the RDA for riboflavin through diet. Thus, to help get to the recommended level of riboflavin, many people need a multivitamin supplement or B-complex tablet.

PANTOTHENIC ACID (VITAMIN B₅)

Pantothenic acid gets its name from the Greek word pantos, which means "everywhere." The meaning of its name should indicate just how prevalent this B vitamin is in plants and animals. At least a small amount of pantothenic acid is present in most of the foods we eat.

Health Benefits

Your body changes most of the pantothenic acid you consume into a substance called coenzyme A, which is required to convert carbohydrates, fats, and some proteins into energy. Pantothenic acid is also necessary for the body to produce hormones and to form hemoglobin and a neurotransmitter called acetylcholine. The adrenal glands also depend upon pantothenic acid for proper functioning, so adequate intake is especially important during times of prolonged stress.

Although some people have claimed that this B vitamin can improve the symptoms associated with rheumatoid arthritis, the limited research in this area has not provided support for this claim.

Who's At Risk For Pantothenic Acid Deficiency?

If you answer yes to any of the following questions, you have an above-average risk of developing a pantothenic acid deficiency.

- *Does your diet consist largely of highly processed foods?* Processing tends to deplete the amount of pantothenic acid in foods.
- *Do you have diabetes?* This disease seems to alter metabolism and increase the excretion of pantothenic acid.
- *Do you drink large amounts of alcohol?* Chronic and excessive use of alcohol can lead to a decrease in the pantothenic acid in your tissues.

The Consequences of a Pantothenic Acid Deficiency

Since the body needs only limited amounts of this nutrient, the risk of a deficiency is minimal. In general, people who are deficient in vitamin B_5 are deficient in all of the other B vitamins as well.

The most common symptoms caused by long-term pantothenic acid deficiency are headaches, nausea, abdominal cramps, fatigue, depression, increased susceptibility to colds, insomnia, and numbness and tingling in the hands and feet.

What Are the Best Food Sources?

Organ meats, salmon, legumes, whole-grain cereals, eggs, and yeast are among the best sources of pantothenic acid. At least some pantothenic acid is present in most foods, however, including chicken, milk, and numerous fruits and vegetables.

DR. ART ULENE'S RECOMMENDATIONS FOR PANTOTHENIC ACID

I recommend a range of 10 to 100 mg of pantothenic acid per day. This compares to the USRDA of 10 mg per day. I advise moving toward the higher levels of my recommendation during times of prolonged stress, and for people who are extremely active physically.

Studies indicate that most people in the U.S. consume 4 to 7 mg of pantothenic acid in their daily diets. To achieve a high intake level, you will probably need to take supplements.

BIOTIN

Biotin gets its name from the Greek word bios, meaning "life." Bacteria in the human intestines often produce enough biotin to meet the body's needs. This B vitamin is also available in common foods.

Health Benefits

Like other members of the B complex family, biotin is important for the metabolism of carbohydrates, fats, and proteins for energy.

Biotin has few substantiated uses in managing medical conditions. Its medicinal use appears to be limited to the treatment of *seborrheic dermatitis*, which is characterized by scaly patches of skin that result from a disorder of oil-secreting glands called sebaceous glands. This condition most often occurs in infants.

Who's At Risk For Biotin Deficiency?

If you answer yes to any of the following questions, you have an above-average risk of developing a biotin deficiency.

- *Do you consume large amounts of raw egg whites?* Egg whites contain an indigestible protein, avidin, which interferes with the body's absorption of biotin. Cooking eggs, however, destroys this protein.

- *Are you pregnant?* Levels of biotin in the blood of pregnant women tend to be lower than levels in non-pregnant women.

- *Are you breast-feeding?* Because biotin is excreted in breast milk, lactating mothers may need to consume more biotin.

- *Do you take anticonvulsant drugs (such as phenytoin, phenobarbital, or carbamazepine)?* Anticonvulsant medications can interfere with the activity of biotin in the body.

The Consequences of a Biotin Deficiency

Because biotin is manufactured by the body and is also found in food sources, deficiencies of this nutrient are rare. Deficiency symptoms include dry, scaly skin and dermatitis, loss of appetite, muscle pain, nausea and vomiting, and neurological problems such as insomnia or depression.

What Are the Best Food Sources?

The best sources of biotin include liver, yeast, soy flour, egg yolks, fish, nuts, chocolate, and cheese.

Biotin is a stable nutrient, and so is not destroyed during cooking.

DR. ART ULENE'S RECOMMENDATION FOR BIOTIN

My recommendation for biotin is 300 mcg per day, which is equal to the USRDA. No toxic side effects have been reported at this dosage.

One recent survey found that most people in the United States consume from 28 to 42 mcg of biotin per day. This is below my recommendation and the USRDA. To raise your intake, you can take biotin as part of many multivitamin preparations or in some B-complex tablets.

VITAMIN C

Over the years, no vitamin has received as much media attention, hype, and hoopla as vitamin C. Thanks in great part to its most prominent and outspoken advocate, Linus Pauling, millions of people religiously consume large amounts of vitamin C hoping it might cure them of everything from the common cold to cancer.

Despite all this attention, the average person isn't sure what to believe about this highly touted nutrient. Furthermore, until recently, most physicians weren't sure what to tell their patients. Research has now provided us with enough information to make recommendations.

Like the B vitamins, vitamin C is water-soluble, meaning that it dissolves in water. Excessive amounts are excreted in the urine.

Health Benefits

Research shows that the vitamin promotes wound healing, helps keep gums healthy, and even reduces the risk of iron-deficiency anemia. Vitamin C also protects against the development of cataracts, cardiovascular disease, and some forms of cancer. Here is what the research shows:

Cancer. A number of large-scale studies have linked a higher vitamin C intake with a reduced risk of cancer, including breast, cervical, lung, and oral cancer. For instance, a study at the University of Toronto and other major medical centers found that women who consumed the most vitamin C were 31 percent less likely to develop breast cancer than women who consumed the least amount of the vitamin. In a study lasting 20 years in Finland, nonsmokers who took the lowest levels of vitamin C were three times more likely to develop lung cancer than those who consumed the highest levels of the nutrient.

Cardiovascular Disease. Some studies have shown that vitamin C may lower total cholesterol, reduce "bad" LDL cholesterol, and increase "good" HDL cholesterol. A daily intake of 1 to 2 grams of vitamin C has been shown to increase HDL cholesterol levels.

Cataracts. With increasing age, vitamin C levels normally in the front part of the eye begin to decline. As levels of the antioxidant decrease, proteins in the lens of the eye become more susceptible to oxidation. The resulting damage to the lens causes a cataract—a clouding of the lens within the eye. Fortunately, adequate vitamin C intake may protect against cataracts, or at least delay their onset.

The Common Cold. Despite the claims of Linus Pauling and other scientists, no definitive evidence exists that large doses of vitamin C can prevent or cure the common cold. Although many carefully conducted studies have not confirmed that vitamin C can reduce the number of colds, there is some indication that it can help individuals recover more quickly from upper respiratory infections.

Longevity. In a decade-long study by researchers at the University of California, Los Angeles, those men who consumed the most vitamin C (about 150 mg daily) had a 35 percent lower death rate during the ten years than men who consumed the least vitamin C (about 30 mg daily). Women who took in the highest amounts of vitamin C had a 10 percent lower death rate than women who took in the least amounts.

Who's At Risk For Vitamin C Deficiency?

If you answer yes to any of the following questions, you have an above-average risk of developing a vitamin C deficiency.

- *Do you smoke?* Studies show that smokers need at least twice as much vitamin C as nonsmokers, because smoking increases the rate of breakdown of this vitamin.

- *Are you an older person?* Older people often take medications that enhance the breakdown of vitamin C. In addition, many older people have poor dietary habits— sometimes because they are on limited budgets or because they live alone and do not cook much for themselves—that compound the problem. Finally, more vitamin C is required to fully saturate certain tissues, particularly white blood cells, in older people.

- *Do you have diabetes?* Studies show that diabetics have lower blood levels of vitamin C than non-diabetics. These lower blood levels occur because ascorbic acid enters cells via the same protein carrier as glucose. When glucose levels are high, as in individuals with diabetes, glucose rather than ascorbic acid is transported, and ascorbic acid is excreted into the urine at a higher rate.

- *Do you drink a lot of alcohol?* Excessive alcohol consumption may cause vitamin C deficits for many reasons. Some researchers believe that alcohol itself destroys the vitamin, while others believe that another, undefined mechanism may be at work. Few argue about alcohol's effect upon overall nutrition; heavy users tend to replace nutritious, vitamin C-rich foods with alcohol.

- *Are you pregnant or breast-feeding?* When the placenta transports vitamin C to the fetus during pregnancy, the mother's concentration of the vitamin tends to fall. When breast-feeding, a woman loses an average of 18 to 22 mg of vitamin C per day. She should increase her intake accordingly.

- *Are you a chronic user of certain medications?* Aspirin appears to interfere with the body's absorption of vitamin C. Although the effects of birth-control pills upon vitamin C are not understood, they may increase excretion of the vitamin in the urine. Other drugs, including tetracycline, increase the breakdown of vitamin C.

- *Are you exposed to high levels of environmental pollutants?* When pollutants are present, vitamin C is particularly important as an antioxidant. The vitamin is necessary for several enzyme systems that help detoxify pollutants (and drugs) and thus minimize their damaging effects. For this reason, you may need extra vitamin C under such circumstances.

- *Have you recently had surgery?* Immediately after an operation, the stress of surgery may produce physiological changes that lower vitamin C levels in the body.

- *Do you have an infectious disease?* Some infections create physiological changes that result in low levels of vitamin C in the bloodstream.

- *Are you on a faddish, unbalanced diet?* Many weight-loss programs are low in vitamin C.

- *Is your baby drinking a formula diet prepared at home with cow's milk?* Cow's milk contains lower amounts of vitamin C than human milk. Your baby may require supplemental vitamin C if cow's milk is part of his or her diet.

The Consequences of a Vitamin C Deficiency

Vitamin C is plentiful in a wide variety of fruits and vegetables, so serious deficiencies are rare in developed countries. Even mild vitamin C deficiencies are relatively rare, and are usually associated with an illness or lifestyle habit, including smoking, stress, and diabetes. A mild deficiency may produce symptoms such as fatigue, loss of appetite, muscle weakness, and a greater susceptibility to infections.

The classic deficiency disease associated with vitamin C is *scurvy*, which is seldom seen in the U.S., usually occurring only in some bottle-fed infants, in elderly people, and in alcoholics. The symptoms of scurvy include rough, dry, scaly skin; swollen, bleeding gums and loose teeth; hemorrhaging in blood vessels; slow healing of wounds; bone and joint pain; and an increased susceptibility to infections. Anemia is also a common symptom of severe vitamin C deficiency. Other warning signs of scurvy are lethargy, fatigue, and change in personality.

What Are the Best Food Sources?

Vitamin C is widely available in both plant and animal foods. Fruits and vegetables such as green peppers, broccoli, potatoes, leafy green vegetables (spinach and turnips), strawberries, tomatoes, melons, oranges, and other citrus fruits are good sources of vitamin C. More modest levels of the nutrient are found in meat, poultry, fish, and dairy products. Grains do not contain vitamin C.

Note that the vitamin C content of any particular food item can vary, depending on factors such as growing conditions, time in storage, and cooking methods used. Vitamin C is highly unstable in the presence of heat, light, and water. Even chopping food into smaller sections can cause the loss of some vitamin C.

DR. ART ULENE'S RECOMMENDATIONS FOR VITAMIN C

My recommendation for the daily intake of vitamin C is 250 to 500 mg per day, which is about four to eight times higher than the USRDA of 60 mg. No toxic side effects have been reported at the recommended dosage. To consume 500 mg of vitamin C per day through diet alone, you would have to drink five 8-ounce glasses of orange juice or ten 8-ounce glasses of grapefruit juice, for example. Most people find that it is more practical to obtain part of their vitamin C requirements through supplements. In fact, when relying on diet alone, only 62 percent of Americans meet even the RDA for vitamin C, according to recent government statistics.

VITAMIN D

Vitamin D is unlike other vitamins in that the body can manufacture this nutrient. (In fact, for that reason, vitamin D fails to meet the classic definition of a vitamin.) Vitamin D is manufactured in the skin, with ultraviolet light driving the process. With regular exposure to sunlight, most people can manufacture enough of this vitamin to meet all of their needs. People who do not get enough year-round exposure, however, may require dietary D as well. Certain groups, including older people, have difficulty producing vitamin D themselves and may also require dietary and/or supplemental vitamin D.

Health Benefits

Some of the strongest evidence pointing to vitamin D's benefits in the body concerns the nutrient's ability to protect against osteoporosis—thinning of the bones—and the bone fractures that can result from this condition. By maintaining sufficient blood levels of calcium, vitamin D promotes bone mineralization, thereby strengthening the bone. While calcium supplementation is an important defense against osteoporosis, most doctors now urge older female patients to take in adequate amounts of vitamin D as well.

In its active form, vitamin D is also involved in the growth and maturation of cells essential to healthy immune system function. A lesser known function of vitamin D is its role in stimulating the production of insulin, a hormone produced by cells of the pancreas.

Who's At Risk For Vitamin D Deficiency?

If you answer yes to any of the following questions, you (or your child) have an above-average risk of developing a vitamin D deficiency.

- *Are you an older person?* Skin production of vitamin D tends to slow down with age. Studies of older people—particularly older women—show that as many as 75 percent are at marked risk for vitamin D deficiencies.

- *Are you confined indoors and not exposed to sunlight?* With limited sun exposure, your skin will produce a minimal amount of vitamin D, leaving you to rely on diet alone for your vitamin D needs.

- *Do you have kidney or liver disease?* Vitamin D, formed in the skin, must be modified chemically in the kidney and liver before the body can use it. This process can be severely impaired if these organs are diseased.

- *Do you regularly take certain medications such as cholesterol-lowering drugs (cholestyramine or colestipol), mineral oil, or anticonvulsants (phenytoin, phenobarbital, or primidone)?* Cholesterol-lowering agents and mineral oil impair the body's ability to absorb vitamin D. Anticonvulsants cause conversion of the vitamin to an inactive form.

- *Do you drink large amounts of alcohol?* Alcohol appears to reduce blood levels of vitamin D and lower absorption by the intestines.

- *Do you drink fewer than three glasses of milk per day?* Except through fortified dairy products such as milk, it is difficult to get adequate quantities of vitamin D routinely in the diet.

The Consequences of a Vitamin D Deficiency

Two common disorders caused by vitamin D deficiency are *rickets* and *osteomalacia*. Rickets is primarily a childhood disease, and in individuals who have it, their bones soften and become so pliable that they bend. It is rare in most parts of the world today, thanks largely to the availability of foods rich in vitamin D, either naturally or through fortification. Children who are breast-fed for a long time without vitamin D supplementation do have an increased chance of developing this disease, however.

Osteomalacia is similar to rickets, involving a softening of the bones.

What Are the Best Food Sources?

Although some foods naturally contain vitamin D—including eggs, butter, oily fish (salmon, herring, and sardines), liver, and cod liver oil—most dietary vitamin D comes from foods that have been fortified. Cow's milk, for example, is usually fortified with vitamin D and is the primary source of dietary vitamin D for children. Infant formula is also fortified with vitamin D. (Breast milk contains little D.) Other commonly fortified foods include margarine and ready-to-eat breakfast cereals.

Plants are not good sources of vitamin D. Green leafy vegetables, for example, contain only small amounts of this vitamin.

Vitamin D is a remarkably stable nutrient; little of it is lost during cooking and storage.

DR. ART ULENE'S RECOMMENDATION FOR VITAMIN D

My recommendation for vitamin D is 400 IU per day. This is equal to the USRDA. No toxic side effects have been reported at this dosage.

It is possible to consume 400 IU of vitamin D per day in your diet, but many people do not do so, partly because there are few vitamin D-rich foods. Most people find that they need to supplement their dietary intake with a vitamin D capsule each day, no matter how much sun exposure they feel they get.

VITAMIN E

Vitamin E actually consists of several fat-soluble compounds that fall into two distinct categories: the *tocopherols* and the *tocotrienols*. The tocopherols are the more active of the two groups, and in particular, alpha-tocopherol is the most potent form and its name is often used interchangeably with vitamin E.

Health Benefits

Studies have suggested that vitamin E may have positive effects in protecting against cardiovascular disease, cataracts, and cancer. It can help strengthen the immune system, and may prove useful in Alzheimer's and Parkinson's diseases.

For example, vitamin E's protective benefits in cardiovascular disease appear to be related to its ability to prevent the oxidation of low-density lipoprotein (LDL) cholesterol, which can contribute to atherosclerosis or hardening of the arteries.

Major studies are now underway, evaluating the effectiveness of vitamin E in preventing Alzheimer's disease. A study at Columbia University's College of Physicians and Surgeons suggested that the progression of Alzheimer's disease can be slowed significantly with high daily doses of vitamin E.

Who's At Risk For Vitamin E Deficiency?

If you answer yes to any of the following questions, you (or your baby) have an above-average risk of developing a vitamin E deficiency.

- *Do you have any of the following chronic illnesses: cystic fibrosis, pancreatitis, biliary cirrhosis, or Crohn's disease?* These illnesses can produce vitamin E deficiencies, particularly when they interfere with absorption of fat from the intestines. In general, however, this poor absorption must persist for five to ten years before signs of a deficiency occur.

- *Is your diet high in polyunsaturated fatty acids (found in corn, safflower, and sunflower oil)?* Vitamin E protects these unsaturated fats from oxidation. When you consume more of them, you need extra vitamin E to maintain the protective role.

- *Are you on a weight-loss (e.g., low-fat, low-calorie) diet?* Inadequate amounts of vitamin E might be consumed while dieting.

- *Do you take certain medications that interfere with vitamin E absorption?* Most commonly, these deficits occur with mineral oil and particular anticholesterol drugs such as cholestyramine and colestipol, when they are taken for long periods of time.

- *Do you smoke cigarettes?* Smoking increases the likelihood of vitamin E insufficiency.

- *Are you exposed to air pollution?* Living in a community with high levels of smog and other environmental pollutants can increase the need for vitamin E.

- *Are you pregnant or breast-feeding?* Extra vitamin E is necessary to ensure proper fetal growth. The RDAs advise a 25 percent increase of this vitamin during pregnancy. Women who are nursing should increase the dose even more.

- *Was your baby born prematurely, with a low birth weight?* A preterm infant may have difficulty absorbing vitamin E and may also have low amounts of the vitamin stored in the liver.

The Consequences of a Vitamin E Deficiency

Vitamin E is common in most diets, and as a result, severe vitamin E deficiencies are rare in the U.S. Reserves of this nutrient are also stored in the tissues of the body.

When a vitamin E deficiency does occur, it can interfere with several body functions, including those related to the reproductive and nervous system, and it may also damage muscle tissues. Common symptoms are a loss of appetite, anemia, mild gastrointestinal distress (such as nausea), eye problems (including cataracts and disorders of the retina), and impairment of the reproductive system (e.g., decreased fertility, an increased risk of miscarriage).

What Are the Best Food Sources?

Vitamin E is available in both animal and plant products. As a rule, plant products contain more vitamin E than animal products do. In addition, meats from animals that have diets high in fat may also be good sources of vitamin E, but because of their high fat content, you're better off finding vitamin E in plants.

The best sources of vitamin E are vegetables and seed oils (such as sunflower, soybean, and cottonseed); however, the distribution of vitamin E compounds differs from one type of oil to another. While the vitamin E content of safflower oil is 90 percent alpha-tocopherol (the most biologically active of the vitamin E compounds), for example, corn oil has just 10 percent alpha-tocopherol. Other good sources of vitamin E are green leafy vegetables, liver, whole grains, wheat germ, butter, margarine, egg yolk, and nuts.

DR. ART ULENE'S RECOMMENDATION FOR VITAMIN E

My recommendation for the daily intake of vitamin E is 200 to 400 IU per day, which is many times higher than the USRDA of 30 IU. The higher level is appropriate for anyone with an increased risk of atherosclerosis and coronary heart disease, and for people who have one or more of the risks listed in "Who's At Risk For Vitamin E Deficiency?"

Recent government statistics show that among adult women, only about 26 percent consume the RDA of vitamin E through diet alone, compared to 35 percent of adult men. Practically speaking, it is almost impossible to consume my recommended dose of vitamin E through just your diet. Nearly everyone will find it necessary to obtain part of their vitamin E requirements through supplements.

FOLIC ACID

Folic acid is a B vitamin that is important for the metabolism of amino acids and the synthesis of proteins. These B vitamins are also involved in the synthesis of DNA and RNA, which are the genetic materials contained in all cells. With the help of vitamin B_{12}, folic acid also ensures the proper formation of red blood cells.

Health Benefits

Studies in the 1990s have shown that folic acid can protect against neural tube defects (NTDs), severe birth abnormalities involving the brain and spine. Based on this persuasive research, the U.S. Public Health Service and the American Academy of Pediatrics now advise all women in their child-bearing years to consume at least 0.4 mg of folic acid per day in order to reduce the risk of having a baby with an NTD.

Recent studies also have shown that adequate amounts of folic acid can reduce levels of homocysteine, an amino acid that increases the risk of coronary disease and stroke. Supplementation with folic acid may also protect against cervical dysplasia in women with low blood levels of the vitamin. (Cervical dysplasia is an abnormal growth of cervical tissues that is considered precancerous.)

Who's At Risk For Folic Acid Deficiency?

If you answer yes to any of the following questions, you have an above-average risk of developing a folic acid deficiency.

- *Are you pregnant?* Pregnant women frequently have folic acid deficiencies if their diets are not monitored carefully. Because the fetus draws folic acid from its mother to promote its own cell division and growth, the mother is at high risk. All pregnant women should have prescriptions for folic acid supplements.

- *Are you breast-feeding?* Because folic acid is lost in breast milk, the RDA for women in the first six months of nursing is for 100 additional mcg of folic acid per day; thereafter, according to the RDAs, nursing women should take an extra 80 mcg of folic acid.

- *Do you consume large amounts of alcohol?* The diets of people who drink excessive amounts of alcohol tend to be low in folic acid. In addition, alcohol appears to interfere with folic acid absorption.

- *Do you use medications such as trimethoprim (for urinary tract infections), anticonvulsants, or birth-control pills?* In particular, anticonvulsant medication such as phenytoin, phenobarbital, and primidone can interfere with the absorption of folic acid.

- *Do you have a malignancy?* Because cancer cells replicate quickly, they use up a lot of folic acid and cause deficiencies.

- *Do you have another nutrient deficiency—particularly of vitamin B_{12}—whose symptoms can mimic those of a folic acid deficiency?* Vitamin B_{12} is needed for the body to properly metabolize and use folic acid.

The Consequences of a Folic Acid Deficiency

A deficiency of folic acid produces a variety of symptoms, including digestive disturbances, sore tongue, fatigue, pallor, memory problems, and paranoia. Deficiency can also cause a form of anemia characterized by malformed, oversized red blood cells, and is associated with symptoms such as headaches, heart palpitations, weakness, and irritability.

What Are the Best Food Sources?

Folic acid is present in green leafy vegetables, oranges, legumes, nuts, liver and other organ meats, and whole-wheat bread and other whole-wheat products. Some fortified, ready-to-eat cereals also contain folic acid.

Folic acid is water-soluble and sensitive to heat. Up to 50 percent of folic acid in foods may be lost in processing and cooking. Losses can also occur if foods are stored where they are exposed to bright light.

DR. ART ULENE'S RECOMMENDATION FOR FOLIC ACID

My recommendation for the daily intake of folic acid is 400 mcg per day, which equals the USRDA. Research suggests that this dosage may reduce the risk of congenital birth defects in children born to women who consume it; it might also lower your risk of coronary disease. No toxic side effects have been reported at this dosage.

Recent statistics from the government's Continuing Survey of Food Intakes by Individuals showed that only 53 percent of women and 68 percent of men consumed the RDA of folic acid through diet alone. Depending on the quality of your diet, you may need to obtain part of your folic acid requirements through supplements.

VITAMIN K

Vitamin K plays a key role in some of the body's most important functions, including blood clotting.

Health Benefits

Vitamin K is a crucial component in the synthesis of proteins involved in blood coagulation or clotting. The liver uses vitamin K to manufacture prothrombin, which is an important blood-clotting factor.

There is also evidence that vitamin K is necessary for proper bone formation. It helps the protein osteocalcin crystallize calcium in the bones, thereby promoting hardening of the bones.

Who's At Risk For Vitamin K Deficiency?

If you answer yes to any of the following questions, you (or your baby) have an above-average risk of developing a vitamin K deficiency.

- *Do you have a chronic illness (particularly a liver disease) or a disorder that interferes with the absorption of fats (such as ulcerative colitis, sprue, or Crohn's disease)?* These diseases can impair the body's ability to absorb and store vitamin K.

- *Are you a chronic user of mineral oil, anticholesterol drugs, or antibiotics?* The non-absorbable fats of mineral oil attach to vitamin K and carry it out of the body. Some anticholesterol drugs (cholestyramine and colestipol) inhibit absorption of vitamin K. Certain antibiotics, including tetracycline, neomycin, and cephalosporins, suppress bacterial production of vitamin K.

- *Is your newborn breast-fed?* Because human milk is a poor source of vitamin K, breast-fed infants are more prone to deficiencies than infants fed fortified formula.

The Consequences of a Vitamin K Deficiency

Vitamin K is found in a wide variety of foods, and thus deficiencies are rare. This vitamin can also be manufactured naturally by intestinal bacteria. Some people, however, are prone to deficits, such as those who use antibiotics, which can destroy the vitamin-manufacturing bacteria in the intestines.

Symptoms of vitamin K deficiency include abnormal blood clotting and an increased tendency to bleed. Individuals who are deficient in this vitamin may experience nosebleeds, as well as bleeding in the gastrointestinal and urinary tracts.

What Are the Best Food Sources?

Bacteria in our intestines manufacture approximately half of the vitamin K we need. We must obtain the rest from our diets.

Spinach and other dark green leafy vegetables are among the best food sources of vitamin K. Significant amounts are also found in meat, milk and other dairy products, eggs, breakfast cereals, and fruits.

Vitamin K is not soluble in water and is quite resistant to heat during cooking. Exposure to light can destroy it, however.

DR. ART ULENE'S RECOMMENDATION FOR VITAMIN K

My recommendation for the intake of vitamin K is 120 mcg per day, which is 50 percent more than the USRDA (at 80 mcg). No toxic side effects have been reported at this dosage.

Through diet, most people consume vitamin K in amounts that meet or exceed my recommendation.

APPENDIX: MINERALS

CALCIUM

Calcium, the most abundant mineral in the human body, makes up about two percent of your body weight. About 99 percent of that calcium is in the bones and teeth; the rest is in tissues and in the body fluids that bathe the cells. In order for your body to absorb the calcium from your diet and make use of it, you also need sufficient amounts of vitamin D.

A mechanism built into your body keeps the levels of calcium in your blood balanced—at sufficient but not excessive amounts. When calcium levels begin to rise too high, the thyroid manufactures a hormone called calcitonin, which draws excess calcium from the blood and deposits it in the bones; urine and feces also carry extra calcium out of the body. Conversely, when calcium levels dip too low, the parathyroid produces a hormone that pulls stored calcium from the bones and sends it to the blood. If the latter process goes on for too long, the bones are depleted of the calcium they need and become thin and weak.

Health Benefits

Eating a calcium-rich diet during the first four decades of life is important in preventing osteoporosis, because it builds bones to their maximum potential before bone mass begins to decrease. After the age of forty, adequate calcium intake is still important, but it will have less of an impact on bone mass and strength than it did earlier in life. While high calcium intake later in life will slow the rate of bone loss, it will not stop the process completely or reverse the damage that has occurred.

Calcium also plays an important role in maintaining normal cardiovascular function. This seems to be due, in part, to its effect on blood pressure. Recent studies have shown that calcium supplements can reduce blood pressure in some people, at least over the short term.

Some research has indicated that high calcium intake may be associated with a reduced risk of colon cancer.

Who's At Risk For Calcium Deficiency?

If you answer yes to any of the following questions, you have an above-average risk of developing a calcium deficiency.

- *Are you an older person?* Older people do not absorb calcium as well as younger adults do and tend not to take in as much calcium to begin with.

- *Do you take diuretics?* Some diuretics change kidney function so that more calcium is lost in urine.

- *Do you exercise frequently?* Perspiration contains calcium. Your levels of this mineral can become depleted if you are extremely active physically—or if you exercise or perform physical labor in very hot weather—and you do not replace the calcium that you lose.

- *Are you on a low-calorie diet?* Dieting often cuts down on the intake of calcium.

- *Is your diet high in protein?* Individuals who eat lots of high-protein foods lose more calcium in the urine than other people do.

- *Is your diet high in fat?* Fats can bind themselves to calcium and interfere with its absorption.

- *Is your diet extremely high in fiber?* Your body has more difficulty absorbing calcium if your diet includes a lot of fiber.

- *Are your vitamin D levels low either because your diet includes too little vitamin D or you have limited exposure to sunlight?* Vitamin D helps the body absorb calcium.

- *Is your diet high in phosphorus?* Foods rich in phosphorus—such as beef, pork, chicken, seafood, cheese, and nuts— may decrease the amount of calcium you absorb.

- *Is your diet high in phytates (found in whole grains) and oxylates (found in spinach, rhubarb, beet greens, and Swiss chard)?* Both of these substances bind with calcium and keep it from being absorbed.

- *Are you pregnant?* A mother supplies an average fetus with about 30 g of calcium over the course of her pregnancy. As a result, the mother may be left with a deficiency.

- *Are you breast-feeding?* Breast milk contains 320 mg of calcium per liter. To replace this, mothers should take more of this mineral while nursing.

- *Are you a smoker?* Smokers have less bone density than nonsmokers. Extra calcium may help to offset this condition.

The Consequences of a Calcium Deficiency

If calcium intake is low for an extended period of time, the mineral is continuously drawn from the bones to keep the calcium concentration in the blood and other organs at a safe level. Eventually, the excessive loss of calcium from the bones can result in the development of osteoporosis.

When calcium deficiency is very severe, the concentration of calcium in the blood may fall low enough to produce symptoms elsewhere in the body. This can include a condition called *tetany*, which causes uncomfortable muscle spasms, and modest increases in blood pressure.

What Are the Best Food Sources?

People in the United States get most of their dietary calcium from milk and milk products such as cheeses. Since milk also contains vitamin D, which helps the body absorb calcium, milk is an especially good choice—whether whole, low-fat, or nonfat. (Milk producers call their product "fortified" because the vitamin D has been added.)

Other good sources of calcium include certain green leafy vegetables (such as broccoli and spinach), beans, nuts, and fish with edible bones (such as sardines and anchovies).

In addition to consuming foods that are naturally rich in calcium, look for products in your supermarket that are calcium-fortified. These include common items such as orange juice, breakfast cereals, and bread.

DR. ART ULENE'S RECOMMENDATION FOR CALCIUM

My recommendation for the daily intake of calcium is 1,500 mg per day, which is higher than the USRDA of 1,000 mg. This recommendation has been chosen to ensure the maximum protection against the development of osteoporosis. No toxic side effects have been reported at this dosage.

You can meet your recommended calcium needs by drinking three glasses of low-fat (1%) milk and eating two 8-ounce servings of low-fat yogurt per day, for example. Most people, however, consume less than my recommendation through diet alone, and according to recent government statistics, only about 22 percent of adult women and 45 percent of adult men consume even the RDA for calcium through diet. You may find it more practical to get part of your calcium through supplements.

IRON

Of all the essential minerals, the most widely known may be iron. The iron you consume passes through the intestines and is absorbed by the bloodstream. About 70 to 80 percent of it ends up in hemoglobin molecules, which give blood its red color and which carry oxygen to cells throughout the body. Some iron also becomes part of a substance called myoglobin, a protein that supplies oxygen to muscle tissue.

Iron is found in other places as well. The liver, the spleen, and bone marrow store it in forms called ferritin and hemosiderin, for instance. But these stores can become depleted if you take too little iron over a long period of time.

Health Benefits

Iron is required by every cell in the body because of the important part it plays in transporting oxygen. Iron is also present in a number of enzymes that are involved in the production of energy.

Iron is a mineral that helps children and adolescents grow. Women require iron for childbearing and for breast-feeding (but lose a lot of the mineral through menstruation).

Who's At Risk For Iron Deficiency?

If you answer yes to any of the following questions, you (or your child) have an above-average risk of developing an iron deficiency.

- *Are you pregnant, or have you recently delivered a baby?* During pregnancy, the fetus and placenta demand a great deal of iron from your body.

- *Are you menstruating?* The average woman loses 15 to 30 mg of iron each month during menstruation; women who bleed heavily or for long periods of time can lose significantly more. For this reason, women who have not yet reached menopause require more iron per day than men or older women.

- *Have you lost blood?* Gastrointestinal bleeding may occur with some conditions, including cancer, hemorrhoids, colitis, and ulcers. Blood loss can also take place during and after surgery or because of an injury. Aspirin or other non-steroidal, anti-inflammatory drugs can also cause chronic bleeding.

- *Do you donate blood regularly?* You lose iron in every pint of blood you donate.

- *Is your diet rich in fiber or tea?* Each of these can interfere with iron absorption.

- *Are you a vegetarian, or do you eat little animal protein?* The body does not absorb the iron in foods in a typical vegetarian diet, including vegetables, beans, and grains, as easily as it does the iron in red meat.

- *Do you consume little vitamin C?* Vitamin C increases absorption of "non-heme" iron—iron found in plant foods. Even if you eat these iron-rich foods, your body will not necessarily absorb the iron from them unless you also consume enough vitamin C.

- *Are you taking antacids?* Antacids can interfere with absorption of iron by the intestines.

- *Is your child young or an adolescent?* Children and teenagers need a lot of iron relative to their body size, partly because they grow so fast during this time.

The Consequences of an Iron Deficiency

Iron deficiency is the single most common nutrient deficiency in the U.S. and the world. Babies and young children who have iron-deficiency anemia are usually pale, irritable and restless, and are often fatigued. Some studies have also shown that iron-deficient children have short attention spans. Adults who have this form of anemia tire easily, and may feel listless and irritable. Other symptoms experienced by iron-deficient adults include: headaches, shortness of breath, decreased appetite, and increased susceptibility to infections and illnesses.

What Are the Best Food Sources?

Popeye may have tried to convince us that spinach is the best food source of iron, but he was wrong. The body can better absorb the iron contained in many other foods.

Red meats (lean cuts) and liver are excellent sources of iron. Because of the high saturated fat and cholesterol contents of these foods, however, it is best not to rely on them too often. Other excellent sources of iron are dark green leafy vegetables. Peas, corn, beans, dried fruits, prunes, and raisins are also good sources. In addition, many foods— including breakfast cereals, breads, and pasta—are fortified with iron.

Remember that your body will absorb iron from some foods better than from others. The best-absorbed iron—heme iron—comes from animal sources and can be found in meats, liver, chicken, and fish. The body does not absorb non-heme iron as well—iron from plant foods such as dried fruits, nuts, beans, and whole grains. Consuming meat, fish, or vitamin C (ascorbic acid) at the same meal with non-heme iron can help absorption. Vegetarians who eat only foods with non-heme iron have an increased chance of developing iron deficiency anemia.

DR. ART ULENE'S RECOMMENDATION FOR IRON

My recommendation for your daily intake of iron is 10 mg per day for men; 15 mg per day for women who are menstruating (in women with heavy menstrual bleeding, the dose can be increased to 20 mg per day); and 10 mg per day for women after menopause. For some people, these recommendations are actually below the USRDA. I've chosen to make these lower recommendations because I'm more concerned about the risk of the average person accumulating too much iron in the body than the risk of individuals without a blood disease developing anemia.

You can consume my recommended levels of iron solely through diet, but not everyone does. You may need an iron supplement if you want to reach the recommended intake for this mineral.

MAGNESIUM

Although every human cell needs magnesium, the average body contains only about 25 grams of it, which is a relatively small quantity. More than half of that is in the bones; the rest is found in places like the teeth, the muscles, the soft tissues, and the blood.

Health Benefits

A growing body of research suggests that a sufficient amount of magnesium in your diet could reduce the risk of heart disease and high blood pressure. Studies have shown, for example, that higher magnesium content in drinking water corresponds to a lower risk of heart disease, probably because magnesium decreases blood pressure. Some research suggests that magnesium supplements could help save the lives of individuals who have just had heart attacks.

Who's At Risk For Magnesium Deficiency?

If you answer yes to any of the following questions, you have an above-average risk of developing a magnesium deficiency.

- *Have you had a lengthy bout of diarrhea or severe vomiting?* Your body loses more magnesium during these episodes.

- *Do you consume large amounts of alcohol?* Magnesium deficiencies are common in alcoholics, primarily because of their poor diets.

- *Do you use diuretics?* Many diuretics cause magnesium to be lost in the urine.

- *Are you pregnant?* According to the Recommended Dietary Allowances, pregnant women should take an additional 20 mg of magnesium per day. This is to meet the needs of the fetus as well as the increased needs of the mother because of her larger body. (Pregnant women gain an average of 30 pounds.)

- *Are you breast-feeding?* Breast milk contains 30 mg of magnesium per liter; to replenish the magnesium lost in nursing, women should consume additional magnesium.

- *Do you have diabetes or kidney disease?* People with these disorders excrete increased amounts of magnesium in the urine.

The Consequences of a Magnesium Deficiency

Severe deficiencies most often occur in individuals whose diets are inadequate or imbalanced, and in people with malabsorption disorders.

The most common symptoms of magnesium deficiency include nausea, muscle weakness or tremors, irritability, loss of appetite, gastrointestinal upset, and rapid heartbeat. Severe deficiency may also cause mental changes, including anxiety and nervousness, confusion, depression, and disorientation.

What Are the Best Food Sources?

Many foods contain generous amounts of magnesium. The richest sources include nuts (particularly cashews and almonds), legumes, leafy green vegetables, and whole-grain cereals. (Note, however, that about 80 percent of the magnesium in cereal grains is lost when the germ and outer layers of the grains are removed during milling—so magnesium may be depleted in processed cereals.)

Except for bananas, fruits tend to be poor sources of magnesium.

DR. ART ULENE'S RECOMMENDATION FOR MAGNESIUM

My recommendation for the daily intake of magnesium is 500 mg per day, which is higher than the USRDA of 400 mg. No toxic side effects have been reported at this dosage, except in people with severe kidney disease (in whom excess levels of magnesium can build up in the body).

While you can, in fact, consume my recommended level of magnesium in your diet, many Americans fall short. (A government survey conducted in the mid-1990s found that only 25 percent of adult women and 33 percent of adult men consume even the RDA for magnesium through their diets.) For that reason, the majority of people need to take magnesium supplements.

SELENIUM

Selenium is a late bloomer among minerals; not until 1979 was it described as a nutrient essential to human health. It is now classified as an antioxidant, with research suggesting that it could play a crucial role in preventing some of the most serious chronic diseases.

Health Benefits

Ongoing research into the effects of selenium has focused on two important areas: cancer and heart disease. With cancer, for example, some research suggests that a deficiency of selenium may contribute to cancer; the mineral might also help prevent cancer. Nevertheless, more research is needed in this area.

Selenium also may provide protection against cardiovascular disease. In a study in Finland, people with very low blood levels of selenium had three times the risk of dying of coronary heart disease, and twice the risk of suffering a heart attack, as people with high levels.

Who's At Risk For Selenium Deficiency?

If you answer yes to any of the following questions, you have an above-average risk of developing a selenium deficiency.

- *Are you pregnant?* Women need extra selenium during pregnancy. According to the RDAs, pregnant women should get an additional 10 mcg of selenium per day.
- *Are you breast-feeding?* Because about 15 to 20 mcg of selenium are lost in every liter of breast milk, the RDAs advise that lactating women consume an additional 20 mcg per day of selenium.
- *Are you under physical or emotional stress?* Animal studies have shown that stress may contribute to selenium deficiencies.

The Consequences of a Selenium Deficiency

When a selenium deficiency occurs, the most obvious symptoms include muscle weakness and discomfort. In serious cases, long-term deficiencies may elevate the risk of developing cardiovascular disease and heart attack, as well as several types of cancers (of the lung, breast, and urinary and gastrointestinal tracts).

What Are the Best Food Sources?

Brazil nuts are the best dietary source of selenium. Seafood, liver, and kidney are also rich in selenium. Other meats tend to be good sources, too, as are milk and egg yolks. Although grains and vegetables (especially mushrooms and onions) can contain substantial amounts of selenium, the precise level depends on the selenium content of the soil in which the crops were grown and the water used to nourish them.

DR. ART ULENE'S RECOMMENDATION FOR SELENIUM

My recommendation for the daily intake of selenium is 200 mcg per day, which is nearly three times as high as the USRDA of 70 mcg. No toxic side effects have been reported at my recommended dosage.

According to one survey, the average adult consumes slightly more selenium than even my recommendation. But because this is an average, many people need a supplement to meet their requirements for selenium.

ZINC

Except for iron, no other trace mineral is as prevalent in the body as zinc. And few have been as highly promoted. You may have heard a lot of claims about zinc, in fact; many myths have flourished around this mineral. Zinc has been touted as a treatment for angina, acne, liver disease, and lack of energy—despite scarce evidence to support any of these claims. Some proponents have even insisted that zinc stimulates sexual potency.

Setting aside the spurious claims, zinc is an essential nutrient that plays important roles in the body. It is present in all of the body's cells, with large amounts in the eyes, liver, bone, skin, hair, and nails.

Health Benefits

Zinc appears to have benefits for the body's disease-fighting immune system. In a study in Belgium, for example, men and women who took zinc supplements had significantly stronger immune function than those who did not take the supplements. At the Cleveland Clinic, individuals with colds who took zinc gluconate lozenges every two hours experienced reductions in their cold symptoms of about three days, compared to people not using the supplements.

Who's At Risk For Zinc Deficiency?

If you answer yes to any of the following questions, you have an above-average risk of developing a zinc deficiency.

- *Is your diet high in fiber?* Dietary fiber can interfere with your body's absorption of zinc. Phytates, found primarily in whole grains and beans, particularly interfere with zinc absorption.

- *Does your diet contain large amounts of phosphorus or iron?* Although the research is not entirely clear on this point, some studies suggest that these minerals may mildly affect the absorption of zinc. Phosphorus-rich foods include milk, meats, fish, poultry, and cheese.

- *Are you a strict vegetarian?* Because the vegetarian diet lacks certain types of food— particularly animal protein and milk products—you may consume less zinc than your body needs.

- *Are you pregnant?* During pregnancy, you need additional zinc to meet the needs of the placenta and the fetus. In animal studies, zinc deficiencies have been associated with developmental disorders.

- *Are you breast-feeding?* Breast milk contains about 1.5 mg of zinc per liter; the RDAs advise consuming an additional 7 mg of zinc per day in order to make up for this loss while breast-feeding.
- *Do you drink large amounts of alcohol?* Regular consumption of large amounts of alcohol can accelerate loss of zinc in the urine.
- *Are you an older person?* Some older people have poor diets that are deficient in zinc.

The Consequences of a Zinc Deficiency

Zinc deficiencies produce signs such as reduced immune function and greater vulnerability to infection; poor wound healing; decreases in appetite; an impaired sense of taste and smell; skin rashes; and a loss of hair. If the deficiency is extended, it can produce slow growth in children and delay the beginning of puberty. In pregnant women, it can jeopardize the well-being of the fetus because zinc is crucial to cell division and growth.

What Are the Best Food Sources?

Most of the zinc in the average U.S. diet comes from animal products. The best sources of zinc include red meats, liver, and seafood. Egg yolks and milk are also good sources of zinc.

The amount of zinc contained in plants depends to some degree on the soil in which the plants were grown, specifically on zinc concentrations in that soil. In general, the best plant sources include legumes such as black-eyed peas. Although whole grains are also good sources of this mineral, the body does not absorb the zinc from them as well as from other sources.

DR. ART ULENE'S RECOMMENDATION FOR ZINC

My recommendation for the intake of zinc is 15 mg a day. This dosage is equal to the USRDA. It is possible to consume 15 mg of zinc per day through diet, but not every adult does. In recent government surveys, only 26 percent of adult men and women consume the RDA for zinc in their diets. Many people need supplements to attain their zinc goals.

REFERENCES

FAT

Krauss RM, Eckel RH, Howard B, et al. AHA Dietary Guidelines: revision 2000: a statement for healthcare professionals from the Nutrition Committee of the American Heart Association. *Circulation* 2000;102(18):2284-99.

St. Jeor ST, Howard BV, Prewitt TE, et al. Dietary protein and weight reduction: a statement for healthcare professionals from the Nutrition Committee of the Council on Nutrition, Physical Activity, and Metabolism of the American Heart Association. *Circulation* 2001;104(15):1869-74.

IMPROVING YOUR FLEXIBILITY

Alter MJ. *Sports Stretch* (Human Kinetics, 1998)

Anderson B. *Stretching* (Shelter Publications, 2000)

Anderson B. *Stretching at Your Computer or Desk* (Shelter Publications, 2000)

AEROBIC EXERCISE

Paffenbarger RS, Hyde RT, Wing AL, et al. Physical activity, all-cause mortality, and longevity of college alumni. *N Engl J Med* 1986;314:605-13.

STRENGTH TRAINING

Nelson ME, Fiatarone MA, Morganti CM, et al. Effects of high-intensity strength training on multiple risk factors for osteoporotic fractures. A randomized controlled trial. *JAMA* 1994;272(24):1909-14.

Treuth MS, Ryan AS, Pratley RE, et al. Effects of strength training on total and regional body composition in older men. *J Appl Physiol* 1994;77(2):614-20.

VITAMINS

Albanes D, Heinonen OP, Taylor PR, et al. Alpha-tocopherol and beta-carotene supplements and lung cancer incidence in the alpha-tocopherol, beta-carotene cancer prevention study: effects of base-line characteristics and study compliance. *J Natl Cancer Institute* 1996;88(21):1560-70.

Cheung MC, Zhao X, Chait A, et al. Antioxidant supplements block the response of HDL to simvastatin-niacin therapy in patients with coronary artery disease and low HDL. *Arterioscler Thromb Vasc Biol* 2001;21:1320-6.

Enns CW, Goldman JD, Cook A. Trends in food and nutrient intakes by adults: NFCS 1977-78, CSFII 1989-91, and CSFII *1994-95. Family Economics and Nutrition Review* 1997;10:2-15.

Harman D. Prolongation of life: role of free radical reactions in aging. *J Am Geriatr Soc* 1969;17(8):721-35.

Jampol LM. Antioxidants, zinc and age-related macular degeneration: results and recommendations. *Arch Ophthalm* 2001;119(10):1417-36.

Omenn GS, Goodman GE, Thornquist MD, et al. Effects of a combination of beta carotene and vitamin A on lung cancer and cardiovascular disease. *N Engl J Med* 1996;334(18):1150-5.

Omenn GS, Goodman GE, Thornquist MD, et al. Risk factors for lung cancer and for intervention effects in CARET, the Beta-Carotene and Retinol Efficacy Trial. *J Natl Cancer Inst* 1996;88(21):1550-9.

U.S. Department of Agriculture. Continuous Survey of Food Intakes by Individuals (CSFII) 1994-96, 1998. Beltsville, MD: Beltsville Human Nutrition Research Center, 2000.

MINERALS
U.S. Department of Agriculture. Continuous Survey of Food Intakes by Individuals (CSFII) 1994-96,1998. Beltsville, MD: Beltsville Human Nutrition Research Center, 2000.

CHOLESTEROL
Appel LJ, Miller ER, Jee SH, Stolzenberg-Solomon R, et al. Effect of dietary patterns on serum homocysteine: results of a randomized, controlled feeding study. *Circulation* 2000;102(8):852-7.

Blankenhorn DH, Nessim SA, Johnson RL, et al. Beneficial effects of combined colestipol-niacin therapy on coronary atherosclerosis and coronary venous bypass grafts. *JAMA* 1987;257:3233-40.

Boushey CJ, Beresford SA, Omenn GS, et al. A quantitative assessment of plasma homocysteine as a risk factor for vascular disease. Probable benefits of increasing folic acid intake. *JAMA* 1995;274(13):1049-57.

Brown BG, Zhao XQ, Chait A, et al. Simvastatin and niacin, antioxidant vitamins, or the combination for the prevention of coronary disease. *N Engl J Med* 2001;345(22):1583-92.

Castelli WP, Garrison RJ, Wilson PW, et al. Incidence of coronary heart disease and lipoprotein cholesterol levels – the Framingham Study. *JAMA* 1986;256(20):2835-38.

De Roos NM, Bots ML, Katan MB. Replacement of dietary saturated fatty acids by trans fatty acids lowers serum HDL cholesterol and impairs endothelial function in healthy men and women. *Arterioscler Thromb Vasc Biol* 2001;21(7):1233-7.

Expert Panel on Detection, Evaluation and Treatment of High Blood Cholesterol in Adults. Executive Summary of the Third Report of the National Cholesterol Education Program (NCEP) Expert Panel on Detection, Evaluation, and Treatment of High Blood Cholesterol in Adults (Adult Treatment Panel III). *JAMA* 2001;285(19)2486-97.

Frick MH, Elo O, Haapa K, et al. Helsinki Heart Study: primary-prevention trial with gemfibrozil in middle-aged men with dyslipidemia. Safety of treatment, changes in risk factors, and incidence of coronary heart disease. *N Engl J Med* 1987;317(20):1237-45.

Krauss RM, Eckel RH, Howard B, et al. AHA Dietary Guidelines: revision 2000: a statement for healthcare professionals from the Nutrition Committee of the American Heart Association. *Circulation* 2000;102(18):2284-99.

Stamler J, Wentworth D, Neaton JD. Is relationship between serum cholesterol and risk of premature death from coronary heart disease continuous and graded? *JAMA* 1986;256(20):2823-28.

SALT
Elliott P, Stamler J, Nichols R, et al. Intersalt revisited: further analysis of 24 hour sodium excretion and blood pressure within and across populations. Intersalt Cooperative Research Group. *BMJ* 1996;312(7041):1249-53.

Midgley JP, Matthew AG, Greenwood CM, et al. Effect of reduced dietary sodium on blood pressure: a meta-analysis of randomized controlled trials. *JAMA* 1996;275(20):1590-7.

The Trials of Hypertension Prevention Collaborative Research Group. Effects of weight loss and sodium reduction intervention on blood pressure and hypertension incidence in overweight people with high-normal blood pressure. The Trials of Hypertension Prevention, phase II. *Arch Intern Med* 1997;157(6):657-67.

Vasan RS, Larson MG, Leip EP, et al. Impact of high-normal blood pressure on the risk of cardiovascular disease. *N Engl J Med* 2001;345(18):1291-7.

ALCOHOL & ALCOHOL ABUSE
Fuchs CS, Stampfer MJ, Colditz GA, et al. Alcohol consumption and mortality among women. *N Engl J Med* 1995;332(19):1245-50.

FIBER
Alberts DS, Martinez ME, Roe DJ, et al. Lack of effect of a high-fiber cereal supplement on the recurrence of colorectal adenomas. *N Engl J Med* 2000;342(16):1156-1162.

Giovannucci E, Stampfer MJ, Colditz G, et al. Relationship of diet to risk of colorectal adenoma in men. *J Natl Cancer Inst* 1992;84(2):74-5.

Rimm EB, Ascherio A, Giovannucci E, et al. Vegetable, fruit, and cereal fiber intake and risk of coronary heart disease among men. *JAMA* 1996;275(6):447-51.

Schatzkin A, Lanza E, Corle D, et al. Lack of effect of a low-fat, high-fiber diet on the recurrence of colorectal adenomas. *N Engl J Med* 2000;342(16):1149-1155.

Smigel K. Fewer colon polyps found in men with high-fiber, low-fat diets. *J Natl Cancer Inst* 1992;84(2):80-1.

Wolk A, Manson JE, Stampfer MJ, et al. Long-term intake of dietary fiber and decreased risk of coronary heart disease among women. *JAMA* 1999;281:1998-2004.

ANGER
Kawachi I, Sparrow D, Spiro A, et al. A prospective study of anger and coronary heart disease. The Normative Aging Study. *Circulation* 1996;94(9):2090-5.

SOCIAL CONNECTIONS & ALTRUISM
Berkman L, Breslow L. *Health and Ways of Living: The Alameda County Study.* New York: Oxford University Press, 1983.

Case RB, Moss AJ, Case N, et al. Living alone after myocardial infarction. Impact on prognosis. *JAMA* 1992;267(4):515-9.

Davis MA, Murphy SP, Neuhaus JM, et al. Living arrangements and dietary quality of older U.S. adults. *J Am Diet Assoc* 1990;90(12):1667-72.

Friedmann E, Katcher AH, Lynch JJ, et al. Animal companions and one-year survival of patients after discharge from a coronary care unit. *Public Health Rep* 1980(4):307-12.

Kiecolt-Glaser JK, Malarkey WB, Chee M, et al. *Psychosom Med* 1993;55(5):395-409.

Reynolds P, Kaplan GA. Social connections and risk for cancer: prospective evidence from the Alameda County Study. *Behavioral Medicine* 1990;16(3):101-10.

Seeman TE, Lusignolo TM, Albert M, et al. Social relationships, social support, and patterns of cognitive aging in healthy, high-functioning older adults: MacArthur studies of successful aging. *Health Psychol* 2001;20(4):243-55.

Siegel JM. Stressful life events and use of physician services among the elderly: the moderating role of pet ownership. *J Pers Soc Psychol* 1990;58(6):1081-6.

Spiegel D, Bloom JR, Kraemer HC, et al. Effect of psychosocial treatment on survival of patients with metastatic breast cancer. *The Lancet* 1989:ii:888-91.

HOW TO GET A GOOD NIGHT'S SLEEP
Belloc NB, Breslow L. Relationship of physical health status and health practices. *Prev Med* 1972;1(3):409-21.

SCREENING TESTS
Expert Panel on Detection, Evaluation and Treatment of High Blood Cholesterol in Adults. Executive Summary of the Third Report of the National Cholesterol Education Program (NCEP) Expert Panel on Detection, Evaluation, and Treatment of High Blood Cholesterol in Adults (Adult Treatment Panel III). *JAMA* 2001;285(19)2486-97.

Frame PS, Berg AO, Wolff S. U.S. Preventive Services Task Force: highlights of the 1996 report. *Am Fam Physician* 1997;55(2):567-76,581-2.

Smith RA, Cokknides V, von Eschenbach AC, Levin B, et al. American Cancer Society guidelines for the early detection of cancer. *CA Cancer J Clin* 2002;52(1):8 22.

ADULTS NEED IMMUNIZATIONS, TOO
Centers for Disease Control, Public Health Emergency Preparedness and Response (www.bt.cdc.gov).

U.S. Preventive Services Task Force. *Guide to Clinical Preventive Services* (2nd edition). Washington, DC: Office of Disease Prevention and Health Promotion, U.S. Government Printing Office, 1996.

U.S. Preventive Services Task Force. Guide to Clinical Preventive Services (3rd edition, 2000-2002). Washington, DC: Office of Disease Prevention and Health Promotion, 2002. Web site: www.ahcpr.gov.

INDEX